Minimally Invasive
Procedures in

UROLOGY

edited by

Steven A. Kaplan
Alan W. Partin
Anthony J. Atala

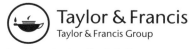

Taylor & Francis
Taylor & Francis Group

Boca Raton   London   New York   Singapore

Published in 2005 by
Taylor & Francis Group
6000 Broken Sound Parkway NW
Boca Raton, FL 33487-2742

© 2005 by Taylor & Francis Group

No claim to original U.S. Government works
Printed in the United States of America on acid-free paper
10 9 8 7 6 5 4 3 2 1

International Standard Book Number-10: 0-8247-2868-8 (Hardcover)
International Standard Book Number-13: 978-0-8247-2868-8 (Hardcover)

Library of Congress Cataloging-in-Publication Data is available.

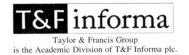

Taylor & Francis Group
is the Academic Division of T&F Informa plc.

Visit the Taylor & Francis Web site at
http://www.taylorandfrancis.com

Preface

The paradigm for treating urologic conditions has undergone a sea of change during the past decade. Guided by new research, the approval of novel pharmaceutical and minimally invasive therapies, and the economics of healthcare financing, physicians have altered their approach to patient care in distinct ways. This evolution in thinking continues today. Indeed, as novel therapeutic modalities become available, as new connections between procedures and outcomes become identified, and as we learn which baseline parameters best predict treatment response in particular patient populations, the therapeutic paradigm is likely to evolve, and progress, still further.

This book is designed to give the reader an up to date review of new techniques and therapeutic alternatives in urology. Specifically, the minimally invasive approach to various disease processes is emphasized. As our population ages and the need to safely and effectively address important quality of life disorders such as erectile dysfunction, voiding dysfunction, and stone disease as well as urologic cancers, we need to be adept at delivering these new technologies to our patients. It is our hope that the techniques described herein will be a good start toward that endeavor.

Steven A. Kaplan
Alan W. Partin
Anthony J. Atala

Contents

Contributors

Clément-Claude Abbou *Service d'Urologie, Centre Hospitalier Universitaire Henri Mondor, Créteil, France.*

David M. Albala *Department of Urology and Radiology, Loyola University Stritch School of Medicine, Maywood, Illinois, USA.*

K. M. Anson *Department of Urology, St. George's Hospital, London, UK.*

Neil Barber *Department of Urology, St. George's Hospital, London, UK.*

John W. Brock III *Vanderbilt University Medical Center, Nashville, Tennessee, USA.*

Culley C. Carson *Division of Urologic Surgery, University of North Carolina Hospitals, Chapel Hill, North Carolina, USA.*

Judy Chun *Division of Urologic Surgery, University of North Carolina Hospitals, Chapel Hill, North Carolina, USA.*

David Y. Chan *James Buchanan Brady Urological Institute, Johns Hopkins Medical Institute, Baltimore, Maryland, USA.*

Bob Djavan *Department of Urology, University of Vienna, Vienna, Austria.*

Steven G. Docimo *Department of Pediatric Urology, The University of Pittsburgh School of Medicine, Pittsburgh, Pennsylvania, USA.*

Aubrey Evans *Division of Urologic Surgery, University of North Carolina Hospitals, Chapel Hill, North Carolina, USA.*

Mohamed A. Ghafar *Department of Urology, College of Physicians & Surgeons, Columbia University, New York, New York, USA.*

Keywan Ghawidel   *Department of Urology, University of Vienna, Vienna, Austria.*

Deborah Glassman   *Department of Urology, Jefferson University School of Medicine, Philadelphia, Pennsylvania, USA.*

R. Greenhalgh   *Department of Urology, St. George's Hospital, London, UK.*

András Hoznek   *Service d'Urologie, Centre Hospitalier Universitaire Henri Mondor, Créteil, France.*

Thomas H. S. Hsu   *Department of Urology, Stanford University School of Medicine, Stanford, California, USA.*

Michael J. Hyman   *Department of Urology, Weill Medical College of Cornell University, New York, New York, USA.*

John Kang   *Division of Urologic Surgery, University of North Carolina Hospitals, Chapel Hill, North Carolina, USA.*

Aaron E. Katz   *Department of Urology, College of Physicians & Surgeons, Columbia University, New York, New York, USA.*

Louis R. Kavoussi   *James Buchanan Brady Urological Institute, Johns Hopkins Medical Institute, Baltimore, Maryland, USA.*

R. S. Kirby   *Department of Urology, St. George's Hospital, London, UK.*

Udaya Kumar   *University of Arkansas for Medical Sciences, Little Rock, Arkansas, USA.*

Michael Marberger   *Department of Urology, University of Vienna, Vienna, Austria.*

Shirin Milani   *Department of Urology, University of Vienna, Vienna, Austria.*

Leif E. Olsson   *Service d'Urologie, Centre Hospitalier Universitaire Henri Mondor, Créteil, France.*

Paul K. Pietrow   *Division of Pediatric Urology, Vanderbilt Children's Hospital, Nashville, Tennessee, USA.*

Ronald Rodriguez   *James Buchanan Brady Urological Institute, Johns Hopkins Medical Institute, Baltimore, Maryland, USA.*

Laurent Salomon   *Service d'Urologie, Centre Hospitalier Universitaire Henri Mondor, Créteil, France.*

David B. Samadi   *Service d'Urologie, Centre Hospitalier Universitaire Henri Mondor, Créteil, France.*

Nelson N. Stone   *Departments of Urology and Radiation Oncology, Mount Sinai School of Medicine, New York, New York, USA.*

Richard G. Stock   *Departments of Urology and Radiation Oncology, Mount Sinai School of Medicine, New York, New York, USA.*

Alexis E. Te   *Department of Urology, Weill Medical College of Cornell University, New York, New York, USA.*

Safwat K. Zaki   *Service d'Urologie, Centre Hospitalier Universitaire Henri Mondor, Créteil, France.*

1

Anatomy and Physiology of the Prostate and BPH

R. Greenhalgh and R. S. Kirby

Department of Urology, St. George's Hospital, London, UK

ANATOMY

The prostate is the shape of an inverted pyramid and lies between the urinary bladder and the pelvic floor. The base is the superior surface and lies at the bladder neck, the anterior border forms the posterior wall of the retropubic space and is attached to the pubic bones by the puboprostatic ligaments. The posterior surface is anterior to the rectum and the inferolateral surfaces are surrounded by the pubo-prosticus fibers of the levator ani muscle. The ejaculatory ducts pass through the posterior surface just inferior to the bladder and open into the prostatic urethra about halfway along its length. It is a fibromuscular and glandular organ that surrounds the prostatic urethra, the fibromuscular element being in direct continuity with the detrusor muscle of the bladder. The true capsule of the prostate is a thin layer of connective tissue at the periphery of the gland. This is surrounded by a condensation of pelvic fascia known as the false capsule. The main blood supply is from the prostatic branch of the inferior vesical artery. The venous drainage is via a plexus between the two capsules. Lymph vessels drain to the internal iliac nodes.

The prostate was originally described as having five lobes by Lowsley; this concept is now no longer considered helpful. Today the prostate is better considered, as described by McNeal, as having four distinct zones. The anterior zone comprises 30% of the gland and consists of fibromuscular tissue only. The rest of the gland is glandular and is divided into peripheral, central, and transitional zones (PZ, CZ, and TZ, respectively). The CZ surrounds the ejaculatory ducts and contains large acini with thick fibromuscular trabeculae. The PZ lies inferior to the CZ and has small acini and narrow fibromuscular trabeculae. The TZ comprises two lateral lobes, which come from the posterolateral recesses of the urethral wall. The TZ and periurethral tissue are the site of development of benign prostatic hyperplasia (BPH) (Fig. 1.1).

This hyperplasia results in slow and gradual reduction in the width of the prostatic urethra, causing symptoms of bladder outflow obstruction (Fig. 1.2).

The enlargement of the prostate comprises two elements, diffuse enlargement and nodular hyperplasia. Diffuse enlargement is seen in nearly all prostates and increases after the age of 40 and appears to be a feature of aging.

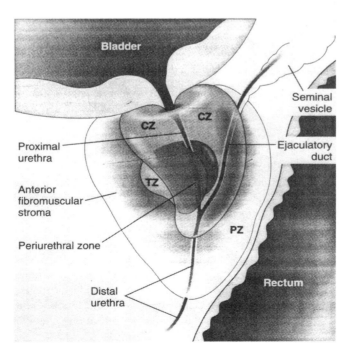

Figure 1.1   From Robbins Pathological Basis of Disease. 6th ed. p. 1025, Fig. 23.16.

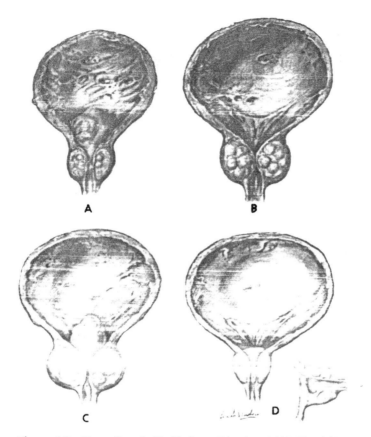

Figure 1.2   From Campbell's Urology. 7th ed. p. 1438, Fig. 46.7.

Nodular hyperplasia is concentrated in the periurethral tissue and in the TZ. Periurethral nodules contain little glandular tissue and are compared mainly of stroma consisting of a pale ground substance with collagen fibers. Glandular TZ hyperplasia is uncommon and consists of large amounts of glandular tissue, which arises from pre-existing ducts (Fig. 1.3).

EMBRYOLOGY

By around day 28 in the developing fetus the urogenital sinus begins to divide the cloaca. By day 44 the rectum and urogenital sinus are separate structures. The primitive urogenital sinus proximal to the mesonephric duct will become the vesicourethral canal; the distal region will become the urogenital sinus proper (Fig. 1.4).

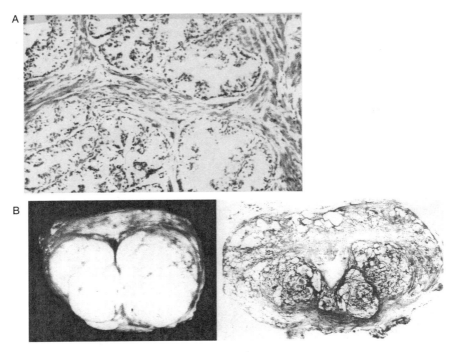

Figure 1.3 (A) Normal prostate histology. (Wolfe. Pathology, Basic and Systemic. 1998. p. 748, Fig. 38.22.) (B) Robbins Pathologic Basis of Disease. 6th ed. p. 1028, Fig. 23.19.

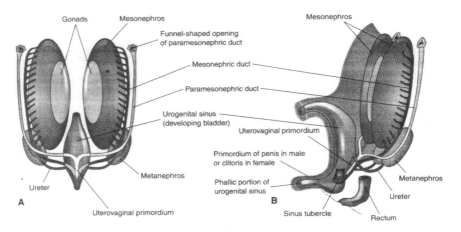

Figure 1.4 The developing human, clinically orientated embryology. (Moore/Pesaud. 6th ed. p. 329, Fig. 13.33.)

During the 12th week of growth prior to the division of the primitive cloaca, the prostate begins its development. Endodermal outgrowths form from the epithelial lining of the prostatic portion of the urogenital sinus and grow into the surrounding mesenchyme. These ducts continue to grow and canalize forming glandular structures. The signal for this development appears to come from the developing testes in the form of testosterone and its more active form 5-alpha reduced dihydrotestosterone, produced by the enzyme 5-alpha reductase locally. The invaginating endodermal cells differentiate in the glandular

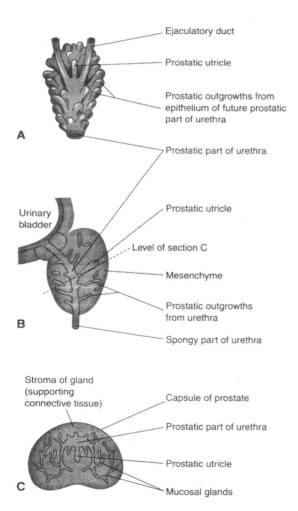

Figure 1.5 The developing human, clinically orientated embryology. (Moore/Pesaud. 6th ed. p. 330, Fig. 13.34.)

epithelium. The stroma and smooth muscle fibers differentiate from the surrounding mesenchyme (Fig. 1.5).

NERVE SUPPLY

Three sets of nerves supply the bladder and urethra: sympathetic T10−L1, parasympathetic S2−4, and somatic innervation via the pudendal nerve S2−4. The main functional innervation to the prostate is through the sympathetic nervous system. It has been postulated that bladder outflow obstruction due to BPH may be related to chronic overactivity of the sympathetic nervous system similar to the overactivity of vasomotor fibers seen in systemic hypertension.

ENDOCRINOLOGY

Prostate growth and development is under the control of the hypothalamopituitary axis. Luteinizing hormone (LH) is released from the pituitary gland when stimulated by LH releasing hormone (LHRH) from the hypothalamus in a pustule manner. Testosterone is released from the Leydig cells of the testes when stimulated by LH (Fig. 1.6).

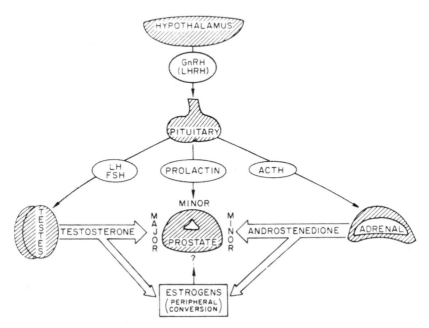

Figure 1.6   From Campbell's Urology. 7th ed. p. 1398, Fig. 45.2.

About 98% of testosterone in the blood is bound to plasma proteins, mainly albumin and sex hormone-binding globulin; this means that only 2% or so of circulating testosterone is available to enter the prostate cells by simple diffusion (Fig. 1.7).

In addition to testicular testosterone, a further 5% of androgens are derived from the adrenal glands under the control of adrenocorticotrophic hormone. Once inside the cell, testosterone is metabolized by a number of prostatic enzymes. More than 90% is converted by 5-alpha reductase on the nuclear membrane to DHT. This is an irreversible process. DHT has a greater affinity for the androgen receptor and is therefore a more potent androgen than testosterone. This binding of the androgen receptor initiates DNA transcription leading to mRNA production for many cytokine molecules including epidermal growth factor, fibroblast growth factor, and platelet derived growth factor. These stimulate prostate cell growth by binding to receptors on the cell membrane of epithelial and stromal cells (Fig. 1.8).

Interestingly, transforming growth factor alpha has been shown to inhibit mitotic activity.

It has been suggested that there is an increase in 5-alpha reductase activity in BPH and an increase in the number of androgen receptors within the nucleus (Fig. 1.9).

Another theory is that there is an imbalance between pro- and anti-mitogenic cytokines.

Experiments in dogs have shown that BPH is associated with a 33% reduction in DNA synthesis, leading to the hypothesis that hyperplasia may

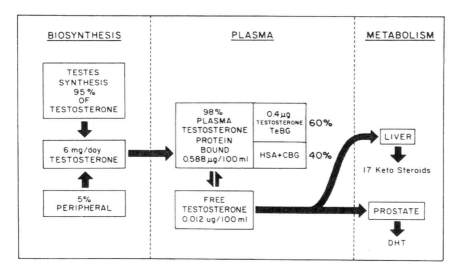

Figure 1.7 From Campbell's Urology. 7th ed. p. 1399, Fig. 45.3.

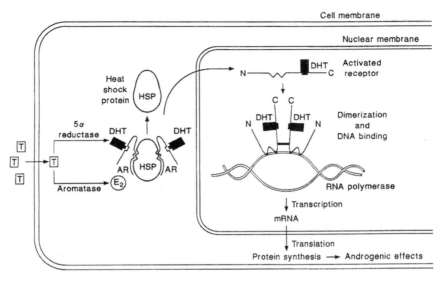

Figure 1.8   From Williams Textbook of Endocrinology. 9th ed. p. 1326, Fig. 29.4.

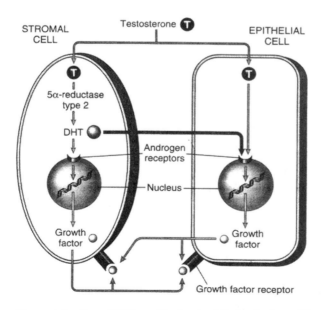

Figure 1.9   From Williams Textbook of Endocrinology. 9th ed. p. 1027, Fig. 23.18.

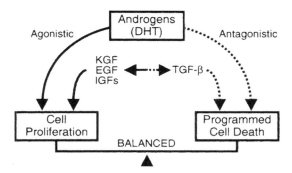

Figure 1.10 From Campbell's Urology, 7th ed. p. 1435, Fig. 46.5.

be due to a decrease in cell death and not an increase in cell replication (Fig. 1.10).

We still have much to learn about the physiological causes of BPH, but the more we discover the more complicated the process appears to be, involving many interacting pathways within the prostate gland.

FURTHER READING

1. Kirby RS, Roerhborn C, McConnell J, Fitzpatrick JM, Boyle P (eds). Textbook of Benign Prostatic Hyperplasia. London: Taylor and Francis, 2004.

Transrectal Ultrasound-Guided Permanent Prostate Seed Implantation: An Updated Technique Using Real-Time Imaging and Intraoperative Dosimetric Adjustment

Nelson N. Stone and Richard G. Stock

Departments of Urology and Radiation Oncology,
Mount Sinai School of Medicine, New York, New York, USA

INTRODUCTION

The treatment of localized prostate cancer now includes a number of minimally invasive modalities that offer similar efficacy as open surgery but with decreased morbidity when compared to standard therapies. Brachytherapy, or prostate seed implantation, is an attractive option for treating T1–T3 prostate cancer because it can be performed in a short period of time with minimal technical difficulty. Studies reporting favorable biochemical freedom from failure rates, low positive prostate biopsy rates, and diminished treatment related morbidity have helped to convince both patients and practitioners that this treatment option should be offered as routinely as radical prostatectomy and external beam irradiation (1–6).

Interstitial irradiation is an attractive form of radiation therapy for localized prostate cancer because it is the most conformal means of delivering the necessary dose. Brachytherapy comes from the Greek "brachy", which means short, because the radiation is delivered over a short distance. The first actual procedures were reported in 1913 by a French urologist (7). This was followed by several investigators who used nonsealed sources of radioactive gold, which were placed into the prostate by an open perineal approach (8). Whitemore et al. (9) developed the first technique for implanting the prostate with permanent sealed sources. Needles were inserted into the prostate through the exposed retropubic space with a free hand technique, using a finger in the rectum to guide their depth. There was no imaging available to determine the relationship of the needles to the prostate or to help guide seed placement.

Holm et al. (10) working in Denmark, began to use transrectal ultrasound to help plan seed placement. Instrumentation included a 5 mHz axial transducer fixed to a stepping device, an applicator, and a crude planning system. This early ultrasound-guided technique was further refined by Blasko et al. (11) who, working in Seattle, developed the modern-day implant technique.

Today there are many variations of the original ultrasound technique, all of which have some common elements that have served to enhance the accuracy of the procedure. These include improvements in ultrasound technology, advances in the dosimetry software programs, changes in the needles and applicators, and alterations in the physical characteristics of the seeds. Along with these improvements have come changes in the technique and its application, which have further improved outcomes for the patients. Recently, the American Brachytherapy Society reviewed the different techniques for permanent source placement and recommended performing the procedure using intraoperative planning with dosimetry feedback (12). This chapter will focus on the real-time technique, which has been enhanced by the addition of intraoperative dosimetric adjustment.

PLANNING FOR THE IMPLANT

One of the differences between the preplan and real-time technique is the ease in planning the implant using the latter method. The urologist should be able perform the ultrasound planning study in the office without the need for anesthesia or concern for significant patient discomfort. The patient is placed in the lateral decubitus position and the transducer is inserted into the rectum. Measurements should be made in two planes using the HWL program of the urologic calculations module. In transverse position the transducer is adjusted so that it images the largest axial slice. Anterior–posterior and lateral (H and W) measurements are taken along the longest axis in each direction. Sagittal imaging is used to determine prostate length. The longest axis is usually measured from the anterior bladder neck to the posterior prostate apex. The most common measurement errors occur with this determination because the probe is not in the midline (it is obliquely rotated) or an intravesical lobe is not appreciated. The patient should not empty his bladder before these measurements, because residual urine facilitates identification of any intravesical tissue. Selecting a true biplanar transducer increases the sizing accuracy. The prostate volume is given to the radiation oncologist who uses a nomogram or look-up table to order the necessary activity for the implant. Isotope-specific nomograms are available from each seed company.

Preparation for seed implant is similar to the preparation for prostate biopsy. Aspirin or nonsteriodal anti-inflammatory medication should be stopped 7–10 days before the procedure. A Fleet enema is given both the night before and the morning of the procedure in order to clean the distal rectum. Antibacterial prophylaxis consists of an oral flouroquinolone with a sip of water 2 h prior to the case. Generally, the antibiotics are continued for 3–5 days after the implant.

IMPLANT PROCEDURE

The patient is brought to the procedure room and given either general or epidural/spinal anesthesia. A urologic X-ray procedure table or general OR C-arm ready table, to allow for fluoroscopy during and after the case, should be used. Once the patient is anesthetized, he is placed in the extended lithotomy position with the buttock brought to the end of the table (Fig. 2.1). The extended lithotomy position is used in order to limit interference by the pubic arch. The rectum should be flushed out several times with water.

A Foley catheter, with 7–10 cc of sterile water in the balloon, is inserted and clamped to maintain between 100 and 150 cc in the bladder. The scrotum is taped to the lower abdomen so that it will be out of the operative field. The probe is placed in the stepping device, which can be attached to the OR table (Fig. 2.2). The table-mounted device, rather than a floor-mounted unit, is preferred because it allows movement of the table during the case. With all of the microadjustment screws and stepper set in their midposition, the probe is advanced into the rectum.

The ultrasound template grid should be aligned so that the lowest row is close to the most posterior part of the gland. The probe can be adjusted up (anterior) or down (posterior) to this position by adjusting the "Y" knob. Next, the prostate should be positioned so that it is in the middle of the grid with both lateral posterior edges of the gland an equal distance from grid points A1 and G1. Imaging is then switched to sagittal and the probe is advanced to view the entire length of the prostate. A tug on the Foley will reveal the position of the anterior bladder neck and the beginning of the bulbar urethra.

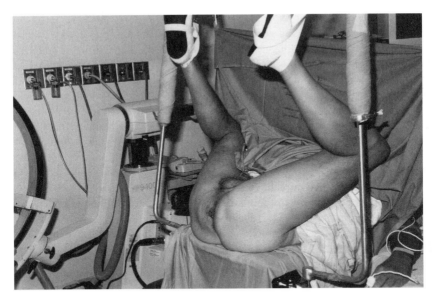

Figure 2.1   Patient is placed in the extended lithotomy position. This position minimizes the risk of pubic arch interference.

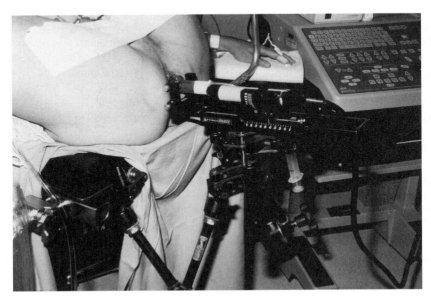

Figure 2.2   Probe is attached to stepper and table-mounted stand and inserted into rectum. Stand has several microadjustment screws to facilitate alignment. (Probe: B&K model 8558, B&K Medical, Marlboro, MA; stand and stepper: BrachyStand, BWM, Sarasota, FL.)

The following anatomical landmarks should be identified: prostate base and apex, presence of intravesical lobe, rectourethralis muscle, urogenital diaphragm, prostatic and bulbar urethra, rectal wall and "plateau", dorsal vein complex, and Santorrini's plexus (Fig. 2.3). The key to accurate seed placement within the gland depends on the development of the intraoperative ultrasound skills necessary to recognize these landmarks.

The rules for intraoperative planning for the real-time implant require that a redetermination of prostate volume using step-section planimetry be performed. The probe is advanced to the base of the gland and the prostate capsule is traced with the track ball. The probe is moved 5 mm caudal, and the process is continued until the apex is reached. This volume is compared to the nomogram and the proper amount of activity is selected for the implant. Of the overall seed activity component, 75% is placed through peripheral needles and 25% through interior needles (13). The implant is divided into two phases, with the peripheral needles placed first using axial imaging for needle insertion and sagittal imaging for seed insertion. The interior needles are placed after determining their correct position with the dosimetry software. The number of peripheral needles is selected by measuring the perimeter of the gland at the largest transverse image. The circumference is rounded up to yield a centimeter length that will equal the number of

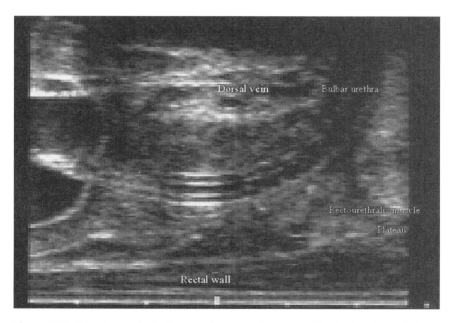

Figure 2.3 Midline sagittal ultrasound image of prostate. Urethral catheter helps to delineate bladder neck and bulbar urethra. Important landmarks include the dorsal vein, rectal wall, rectourethralis muscle, and associated rectal plateau.

peripheral needles required. This process will allow for slightly less than 1 cm spacing between each peripheral needle.

The total number of seeds required is based on the total activity (derived from the nomogram) divided by the activity per seed on the day of the implant. For example, the total activity for a 34 cc gland might be 30 mCi. If the I-125 seeds have an activity of 0.33 mCi, then 90 seeds are required (30/0.33 = 90). Seventy seeds (75% of 90) would be placed through the peripheral needles and 20 through the interior needles. If 14 peripheral needles were required, then each needle would receive five seeds (14 × 5 = 70 peripheral seeds).

The ultrasound probe is placed in transverse imaging and the largest axial image of the prostate is found. The most posterior applicator needles are placed first. These needles are spaced 1 cm apart and should be placed 1–2 mm interior to the capsule (Fig. 2.4). The posterior row of needles should be placed at least 7 mm above the rectal mucosa. The remaining outer needles are next placed. Starting at the 7 o'clock position, each subsequent needle is passed through the outer template so that it ends up approximately 1 cm away from the preceding needle as it appears on the ultrasound image. Keep in mind that the outer template acts only as a guide for needle placement and that the actual location of needles in relationship to one another and the prostate can be determined only from the ultrasound image. Needle placement may require a few passes through different

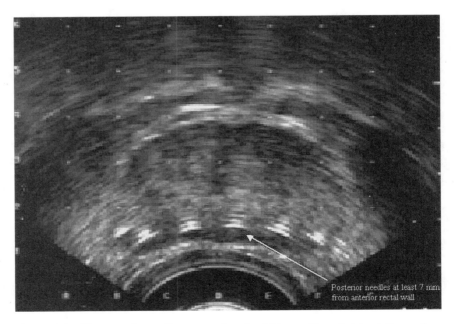

Posterior needles at least 7 mm from anterior rectal wall

Figure 2.4 The posterior applicator needles should be positioned at least 7 mm above the rectal mucosa.

holes in the outer template to find the right position on the ultrasound image. When placing these outer needles, the goal is to keep them as lateral or as peripheral as possible. This will result in the desired dose of radiation covering the prostate with an adequate margin (Fig. 2.5).

Intraoperative dosimetry, generated using the brachytherapy software, allows immediate updates of needle and seed positions, which can be incorporated into the procedure as it progresses. There are several vendors that offer commercial software, which is continually undergoing revision as the procedure moves to a more real-time method. The method described subsequently has been shown to closely represent the results encountered on the postimplant dosimetry studies (14). Once all peripheral needles are placed, the first step of real-time dosimetry is performed. The prostate is contoured from base to apex at 5 mm intervals and the urethra identified by a marker. Each contoured prostate slice containing the peripheral needles is acquired and stored by the treatment planning system. The internal grid of the planning system is superimposed on the grid positions of the acquired ultra sound images. On each acquired prostate slice, the prostate is contoured and the urethral marker circled (Fig. 2.6). In addition, the anterior rectum is outlined (perirectal fat and mucosa). The planning system creates a three-dimensional grid matrix with x-, y-, and z-axes (Fig. 2.7).

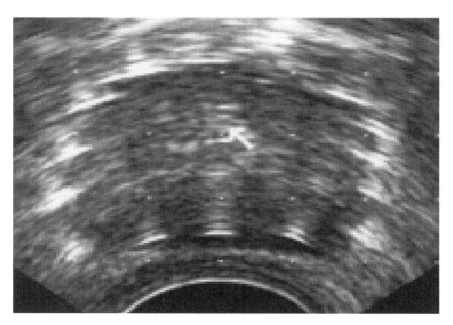

Figure 2.5   All of the peripheral needles have been placed. Needles are spaced <10 mm from each other.

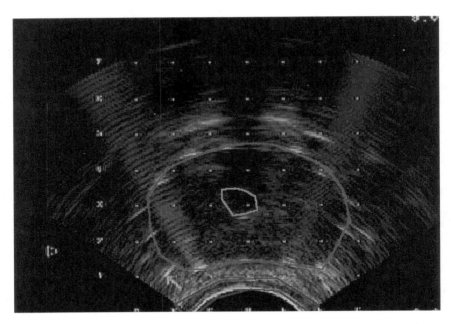

Figure 2.6 (**See color insert following page 150**) Acquired transverse prostate image (red) with peripheral needles in place is outlined on the computer using the dose planning software. The urethra (green) and anterior rectal wall (blue) are also identified in order to calculate radiation doses to these structures. (VariSeed 6.7, Varian Medical Systems, Charlottesville, VA).

After image acquisition the implant procedure begins. The seeds are implanted with a Mick applicator (TP-200, Mick Radionuclear Instruments, Mount Vernon, NY) using sagittal ultrasound imaging as a guide to needle and seed location (Fig. 2.8). The implant is started at the most lateral posterior (7 o'clock) needle. The needle is advanced to the base of the gland and the first seed is placed while observing that the needle is proximal to the prostate capsule at the base. The goal for each row is to place the first seed at the base, the last one at the apex, and intervening seeds (usually two–four) evenly spaced between the two ends of the gland. After finishing the first needle, the probe is rotated a few degrees clockwise and the next lateral–anterior needle is located and implanted. The entire peripheral implant takes ∼20 min. During this time, the physicist works to complete the dosimetric representation of the implant.

The position of the needles in the treatment planning system is determined based on the acquired ultrasound images with the actual implant needles in place. The planning system assumes that the needles run straight and do not deviate. In other words, it assumes that the needles run parallel with the z-axis. Needle positions are identified by the echo-bright flash present on the acquired transverse

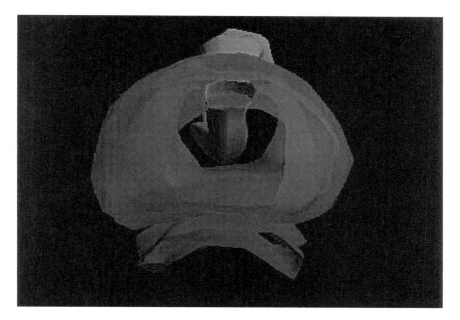

Figure 2.7   (**See color insert**) Three-dimensional reconstruction of prostate prior to seed insertion. Prostate is in red, urethra in green, and rectum in blue.

images. The needle position is first identified by locating the nearest grid position to the needle. This point is dragged to the spot corresponding to the image of the needle on the acquired ultrasound image (Fig. 2.9). The number of peripheral needles identified matches the number of needles actually inserted. The number of seeds implanted per needle is registered onto the real-time planning (RTP) system simultaneously. The location of the seeds in the RTP matrix is determined manually by examining the path of the needle through the transverse captured prostate images. For example, a seed would not be placed on a prostate slice in which the needle clearly lies outside the prostate. Seeds can be placed on any of the 5 mm slices or 2.5 mm above or below any slice. The number of seeds implanted into the peripheral needles on the RTP must match the actual number of seeds implanted in the periphery of the prostate.

The next step involves placing the internal needles. The remaining 25% of the seeds are inserted via these needles. Typically, between six and nine needles are inserted into the interior such that they encompass the periphery of the base and apical slices and are 0.5–1 cm from the urethra. The physicist inserts the needles on the previously acquired images and then places one seed in each needle at the base and apical slices. Starting at the base of the gland, the isodose

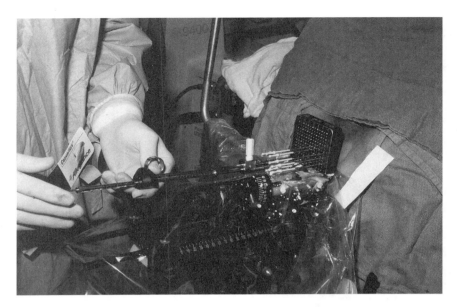

Figure 2.8 Mick applicator is attached to the lateral posterior needle and seeds are inserted working from base to apex. Sagittal ultrasound imaging is used to position seeds, which should be evenly spaced as needle is withdrawn toward the apex.

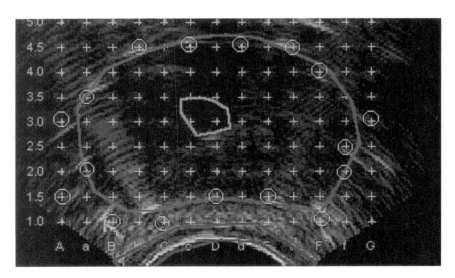

Figure 2.9 (**See color insert**) Needles are positioned first on grid point (top) and then dragged to actual position (bottom) of needle on the acquired ultrasound image.

contours are visualized. Additional seeds can be placed or needle positions adjusted to ensure that the 100% isodose line covers each prostate slice with a margin. The 150% isodose line is also visualized to make sure it does not cover the urethra or extend into the rectum (Fig. 2.10). The physicist can make these adjustments by

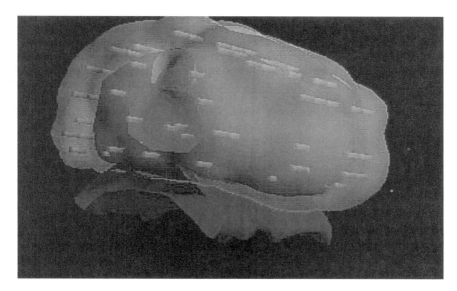

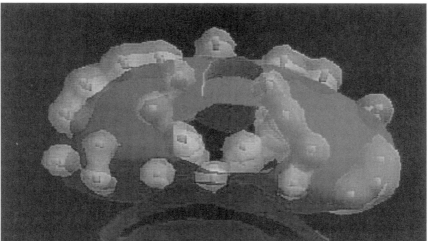

Figure 2.10 (**See color insert**) Three-dimensional image showing 140 Gy dose cloud (yellow) encompassing the prostate (top). The high-dose regions (150% of prescription) are distributed away from the urethra and center of the gland (bottom).

adding or deleting seeds. The physicist then checks the dose volume histogram (DVH) values. The dosing rules to follow are based on prostate-specific antigen (PSA), biopsy, and quality of life (QOL) data (Table 2.1) (15–18). Once the team is satisfied with the plan, the interior needles are inserted accordingly. Seeds are deposited in each needle as indicated by the plan.

A fluoroscopic image should be taken after all seeds have been placed and the implant is completed. Contrast media are injected through the Foley catheter with a little force in order to identify any loose seeds in the bladder (19). If there is any suspicion that seeds may have been deposited in the urinary tract, they can be removed cystoscopically. The ultrasound probe is removed from the rectum, the perineum washed off with sterile saline, and an antibacterial ointment applied to the puncture sites. A dry sterile gauze dressing is placed over the implant site and pressure applied for a few minutes.

POSTIMPLANT GUIDELINES

Patients with large prostates or those with a large median lobe often have difficulty with hesitancy, poor stream, or urinary retention. If the patient is unable to void the next day, it is best to send him home catheterized with a leg bag and wait for the prostatic swelling to subside. Anti-inflammatory medications and alpha blockers often are helpful. If urinary retention persists despite these measures, it is probably safest to place a suprapubic drainage catheter or institute self-catheterization while waiting for the retention to resolve. The prostate gland will eventually shrink 40–50% from the effect of the radiation over time. This will allow resolution of the urinary retention in the majority of the patients. If retention persists, the patient may require surgical intervention. Options include transurethral incision or resection of the obstructing tissue (20). There is very little experience in the use of lasers or vaporizing electrodes in these cases, and until more experience is gained with them, it is probably best to not use them at this time.

In cases of outlet obstruction not relieved with catheterization, transurethral resection of the prostate (TURP) may become necessary. If this procedure is

Table 2.1   Dosing Guidelines for Intraoperative Dosimetric Adjustment

Isotope	Prostate (D_{90})	Urethra (30% of volume)	Rectal volume
I-125	160–180 Gy	<150%	160 Gy to <1.3 cc
Pd-103	124–135 Gy	<150%	124 Gy to < 1.3 cc
pI-125	107 Gy	<150%	107 Gy to <1.3 cc
pPd-103	100 Gy	<150%	100 Gy to <1.3 cc

Note: The dose rules for I-125 are based on PSA, biopsy, and QOL outcome data. The guidelines for Pd-103, partial Pd-103 (pPd-103) and partial I-125 (pI-125) are extrapolated from the iodine data. pI-125 = partial implant.

required, it is preferable to wait for at least three–four half-lives of the isotope to expire (Pd-103: 51 days, I-125: 180 days) so that most of the radiation therapy has been delivered. The urologist should contact the radiation oncologist when planning a TURP so that the remaining activity can be calculated and proper disposal of the radioactive seeds can be planned.

It is not unusual for patients to experience postimplant irritative urinary symptoms. These usually result from mild radiation urethritis while the radiation is being given off from the seeds. Patients with Pd-103 implants tend to experience these earlier and for a shorter duration than those who receive I-125 implants. As with most patients who experience these symptoms due to other causes, antispasmodics or urinary analgesics are often helpful. Similar to patients with interstitial cystitis, patients sometimes experience irritation with certain foods. In such cases a temporary diet restriction of caffeine, spices, acids, and citrate products (fruit juices, tomato sauce, etc.) may be beneficial. In addition, anti-inflammatory medications such as NSAID or low-dose steroids can be used to treat the symptoms caused by the prostate edema associated with radiation therapy. In the majority of cases these symptoms will resolve spontaneously, and the physician's reassurance will go a long way in reducing the patient's anxiety.

The majority of patients should not experience any rectal discomfort following implantation. For complaints of rectal temesmous (recurrent urge to defecate), minor bleeding, or rectal/perineal pain, a course of steroid foam suppositories will often be helpful.

POSTIMPLANT CT-BASED DOSIMETRY

CT-based dosimetry should be performed 1 month after implantation using commercial three-dimensional treatment planning software. CT images of the prostate at 3 mm, abutting slices throughout the implanted area, are collected. On every CT slice, the prostate is contoured, the urethra located, and the rectum identified. DVHs of these structures are generated. The dosimetry values that should be achieved are shown in Table 2.2. The dose delivered to 90% of the prostate volume (D_{90}) is the index most often used to assess the adequacy of the implant.

PROSTATE BRACHYTHERAPY RESULTS

The results of treatment for patients undergoing prostate brachytherapy depend on several variables. Pretreatment patient characteristics, the use of hormonal therapy, the addition of external beam irradiation, and the definition used to define failure all will impact the implant success rates. The best way to evaluate outcomes regarding treatment efficacy is to stratify patients into risk categories. Patients with a PSA ≤ 10 ng/mL, clinical stage T2a or less, and a Gleason score ≤ 6 are considered to be low risk. A PSA between 10 and 15 ng/mL, a Gleason

Table 2.2 Postimplant Dosimetry Results
Should Fall within the Ranges Shown

Implant type	D_{90} (Gy)
I-125	140–180
Pd-103	120–135
partial Pd-103 or I-125	90–110

Note: For monotherapy (full-dose implant, no external beam) the lower-value dose should be achieved in all patients. Patients with D_{90} above the higher value may be at increased risk for early and late morbidity. The partial implant doses are delivered in patients who receive a combination of seed implant and external beam irradiation. It is preferred to perform the implant first so that the dosimetry data are available to make any adjustments in the external beam treatment.

score of 7, or palpable disease involving the entire lobe places the patient in the intermediate risk category. High-risk patients can be defined as those with a PSA > 15 ng/mL, a Gleason score of 8 or higher, or stage $>$T2c. Some also consider patients to be at high risk if they have two or more moderate risk features.

Low-risk patients treated with permanent seed implant have an outcome similar to radical prostatectomy and external beam irradiation. PSA disease-free survival ranges from 50–100% at 5 years to 60–88% at 10–12 years. For intermediate risk patients biochemical control rates of 35–86% (Tables 2.3 and 2.4) (1–6,18,21–27). High-risk patients have poor outcomes when treated with implant alone but an improved result with the addition of hormonal therapy or external beam irradiation (Table 2.5) (21–29).

COMPLICATIONS OF BRACHYTHERAPY

Most patients who undergo seed implantation will experience some degree of acute urinary morbidity. Urinary retention occurs between 1% and 10% of the time and is more common in patients with large prostates or in those with significant urinary symptoms. Gelblum et al. (30) noted a greater risk of obstructive symptoms and urinary retention in patients with prostates larger than 35 cc. Terk et al. (20) reported that the patient's pre-implant international prostate symptom score (IPSS) was the most important predictor of urinary retention. The incidence of retention can be reduced in patients by pretreatment with an alpha blocker prior to the procedure (30). Unresolved urinary retention requires surgical intervention. It is usually safe to perform a TURP 2 months after a Pd-103 and 6 months after an I-125 implant. Postimplant TURP rates range from 0% to 8.3% (2,20,30–32).

Table 2.3 Prostate Brachytherapy PSA Outcomes in Low-Risk Patients

Study	Patient characteristics	Number	Biochemical control (%)	PSA failure definition	Years
Brachman	PSA ≤4	128	85	ASTRO[c]	7
	PSA 4–10	345	74		
Critz[a]	PSA ≤4	50	94	PSA >0.2	5
	PSA 4–10	451	93		
Dattoli	PSA <10, score <7, Stage <T2b	74	93	PSA >1.0	6
Grimm	Low risk: 1986–1987	75	64	ASTRO[c]	10
	Low risk: after 1987	97	88		
Potters	Low risk	NA	88	ASTRO[c]	5
Ragde	Score <7, Stage <T2b	140	60	PSA >0.5	12
Stone[b]	PSA <10	76	95	ASTRO[c]	6

[a]Patients treated with a combination of implant and beam irradiation.
[b]Patients treated with 6 months of hormonal therapy.
[c]American Society of Treating Radiation Oncologists.

Most patients will experience dysuria, frequency, urgency, weak stream, and nocturia. Kleinberg reported nocturia as the most common acute urinary symptom following I-125 implantation. Eighty percent complained of increased urinary symptoms 2 months after the implant, which lasted up to a year in 45%

Table 2.4 Biochemical Control Rates in Intermediate Risk Patients

Study	Patient characteristics	Number	Biochemical control (%)	PSA failure definition	Years
Brachman	PSA 10–20	144	53	ASTRO[g]	7
Critz[a]	PSA 10–20	144	75	PSA >0.2	5
Grado	PSA 10–20	119	72	Two elevations in PSA	5
Grimm	Intermediate risk	22	80[b]	ASTRO[g]	10
		27	35[c]		
Potters	Intermediate risk	NA	81[d]	ASTRO[g]	5
			85[e]		
Stone[f]	PSA 10–20	58	86	ASTRO[g]	6

[a]Patients treated with a combination of implant and beam irradiation.
[b]Patients treated after 1987.
[c]Patients treated prior to 1988.
[d]Implant alone.
[e]Implant plus beam irradiation.
[f]Patients treated with 6 months of hormonal therapy.
[g]American Society of Treating Radiation Oncologists.

Table 2.5 Biochemical Control Rates in High-Risk Patients

Study	Patient characteristics	Number	Biochemical control	PSA failure definition	Years
Brachman[a]	PSA >20	73	33	ASTRO[e]	7
Critz[c]	PSA >20	44	69	PSA >0.2	5
Potters	High risk	NA	74[b] 79[c]	ASTRO[e]	5
Ragde	Stage ≥T2b Score ≥7 PSA >10	82	79	PSA >0.5	12
Stock[d]	High risk	85	81	ASTRO[e]	5
Zeitlin[c]	Stage ≥T2b Score ≥7 PSA >10	67 69 119	76	PSA >0.5	5

[a]Patients treated with implant alone.
[b]Implant alone.
[c]Implant plus beam irradiation.
[d]Patients treated with 9 months of hormonal therapy, implant, and beam irradiation.
[e]American Society of Treating Radiation Oncologists.

(33). Desai et al. (34) found that the mean total IPSS increased from 6 to 14 within a month after implant. It took 12–18 months for symptoms to return to normal. Urinary symptoms were also highly correlated to the radiation dose received by the prostate and urethra. Most studies have found that ~90% of patients will have normalized their urinary complaints by 1 year postimplant (35,36).

Chronic urinary morbidity will occur if the prostatic urethra receives too high a dose of radiation. Complications include irritative voiding symptoms and urethral scarring. Grade 3 Radiation Treatment Oncology Group (RTOG grading) urinary morbidity has been found to occur in 1–3% of the patients (37,38). Stock et al. (39) have shown that this complication is rare if prostate and urethral radiation doses do not exceed the tolerance levels (<150% of prescription delivered to 30% of urethral volume). Urinary obstruction can occur if there is radiation injury to the bladder neck or urethra. Prior prostatic surgery can result in bladder neck contracture following an implant. Surgical correction of these patients has a high likelihood of incontinence. Ragde et al. (40) described this event in 2.5% of his patients who required a urinary diversion as treatment. Placement of seeds around the bulbar urethra can cause a stricture, which has been reported in as many as 12% of the patients (40). This complication most likely occurs when seeds are placed too caudal just anterior to the prostate apex.

Urinary incontinence has been reported in 0–85% of the patients. The higher rates come from studies where patients reported this problem (41).

Chronic urinary incontinence is also rare in patients without a prior history of prostate surgery (TURP) and as high as 85% in men with prior TURP. Incontinence can be minimized by performing a peripheral loaded implant (42).

Rectal damage can also result from a permanent seed implant. Damage can be mild and self-limiting, such as minor occasional bleeding, or severe enough to cause a prostatorectal fistula. Proctitis rates range from 1 to 21.4% (21,23, 42–46). A higher incidence is expected in those patients who receive a combination of seed implant and external beam irradiation. More severe rectal complications such as ulcer (grade 3) or fistula formation (grade 4) have been more commonly reported in patients who have had their rectal bleeding treated by some form of caustic therapy. Theodorescu et al. (7) reported 7 fistulas among 724 men treated with implant alone or in combination with external beam. Six or seven of the patients had their rectal bleeding managed by biopsy and electrocautery (47). Gelblum noted that 50% of the grade 3 rectal complications had an antecedent rectal biopsy and that the biopsied patients took twice as long to heal (46). Most experienced brachytherapists caution patients against biopsy and fulguration of bleeding areas in the anterior rectal wall. Hu and Wallner (48) have shown that most rectal bleeding will resolve spontaneously. It is prudent to caution the patients not to have any rectal procedures performed without getting clearance from the physicians who performed the implant. Recently, Snyder et al. (49) have shown that the volume of rectum treated by the prescription dose is highly correlated to the development of grade 2 proctitis.

Preservation of erectile function occurs in 62–86% of patients who were followed 1–6 years after implantation (2,43,50,51). Men with normal erectile function prior to implantation have a much higher likelihood of maintaining function after implantation than those who present with poor erection capacity (51). High-radiation doses also have a negative impact on sexual function (51).

This chapter has described one of the newer techniques for prostate brachytherapy. It is hoped that many urologists and radiation oncologists will take the opportunity to learn and master it. There is no doubt that there is a relationship between technical expertise and implant quality. The brief review reported here on PSA and QOL outcomes demonstrates a wide range of results, some of which can be explained by how well the implant was performed. Consistent implant quality will result in high cancer cure rates and significant quality of life benefits.

REFERENCES

1. D'Amico AV, Whittington R, Malkowicz SB, Schultz D, Blank K et al. Biochemical outcome after radical prostatectomy, external beam radiation therapy, or interstitial radiation therapy for clinically localized prostate cancer. J Am Med Assoc 1998; 280:969–974.

2. Dattoli MJ, Wallner K, True L, Cash J, Sorace R. Long-term outcomes after treatment with external beam radiation therapy and palladium 103 for patients with higher risk prostate carcinoma: influence of prostatic acid phosphatase. Cancer 2003 Feb 15; 97(4):979–983.

3. Blasko JC, Ragde H, Luse RW et al. Should brachytherapy be considered a therapeutic option in localized prostate cancer? Urol Clin North Am 1996; 23:633–650.

4. Ragde H, Abdel-Aziz AE, Snow PB, Brandt J, Bartolucci AA et al. Ten-year disease free survival after transperineal sonography-guided iodine-125 brachytherapy with or without 45-gray external beam irradiation in the treatment of patients with clinically localized, low to high Gleason grade prostate carcinoma. Cancer 1998; 83:989–1001.

5. Sharkey J, Chovnick SD, Behar RJ, Perez R, Otheguy J et al. Outpatient ultrasound-guided palladium 103 brachytherapy for localized adenocarcinoma of the prostate: a preliminary report of 434 patients. Urology 1998; 51:796–803.

6. Stokes SH, Real JD, Adams PW, Clements JC, Wuertzer BS, Kan W. Transperineal ultrasound-guided radioactive seed implantation for organ-confined carcinoma of the prostate. Int J Radiat Oncol Biol Phys 1997; 37:337–341.

7. Pasteau O, Degrais P. The radium treatment of cancer of the prostate. J Urol (Paris) 1913; 4:341–366.

8. Flocks RH, Kerr HD, Elkins H et al. Treatment of carcinoma of the prostate by interstitial radiation with radioactive gold (Au 198): a preliminary report. J Urol 1952; 68:516–522.

9. Whitmore WF, Hilaris B, Grabstald H. Retropubic implantation of iodine 125 in the treatment of prostate cancer. J Urol 1972; 108:918–920.

10. Holm HH, Pedersen JF, Hansen H, Stroyer I. Transperineal I-125 iodine seed implantation in prostatic cancer guided by transrectal ultrasonography. J Urol 1983; 130:283–286.

11. Blasko JC, Radge H, Schumacher D. Transperineal percutaneous iodine-125 implantation for prostatic carcinoma using transrectal ultrasound and template guidance. Endocurie Hypertherm Oncol 1987; 3:131–139.

12. Nag S, Ciezki JP, Cormack R, Doggett S, DeWyngaert K, Edmundson GK, Stock RG, Stone NN, Yu Y, Zelefsky MJ. Intraoperative planning and evaluation of permanent prostate brachytherapy: report of the American Brachytherapy Society. Int J Radiat Oncol Biol Phys 2001; 51(5):1422–1430.

13. Stone NN, Stock RG, DeWyngaert JK, Tabert A. Prostate brachytherapy: improvements in prostate volume measurements and dose distribution using interactive ultrasound guided implantation and three-dimensional dosimetry. Radiat Oncol Invest 1995; 3:185–195.

14. Stock RG, Stone NN, Lo YC. Intraoperative dosimetric representation of the real-time ultrasound guided prostate implant. Tech Urol 2000; 6:95–98.

15. Merrick G, Butler WM, Dorsey et al. Potential role of various dosimetric quality indicators in prostate brachytherapy. Int J Radiat Oncol Biol Phys 1999; 44:717–724.

16. Stock RG, Stone NN, Lo YC, Malhado N, Kao J, DeWyngaert JK. Post-implant dosimetry for I-125 prostate implants: definitions and factors affecting outcome. Int J Radiat Oncol Biol Phys 2000; 48:899–906.

17. Stock RG, Stone NN, Dalal L, Lo YC. What is the optimal dose for I-125 prostate implants? A dose response analysis of long-term urinary symptoms, biochemical control and post-treatment biopsy. Int J Radiat Oncol Biol Phys 2000; 48(suppl):74.
18. Stock RG, Stone NN, Tabert A, Iannuzzi C, DeWyngaert JK. A dose-response study for I-125 prostate implants. Int J Radiat Oncol Biol Phys 1998; 41:101–108.
19. Stone NN, Stock RG. Dynamic cystography can replace cystoscopy following prostate seed implantation. Tech Urol 2000; 6:112–116.
20. Terk M, Stock RG, Stone NN. Identification of patients at an increased risk for prolonged urinary retention following radioactive seed implantation of the prostate gland. J Urol 1998; 160:1379–1382.
21. Stone NN, Stock RG. Prostate brachytherapy: treatment strategies. J Urol 1999; 162:421–426.
22. Potters L, Cha C, Ashley R, Freeman K, Waldbaum R, Wang X-H, Liebel S. The role of external beam irradiation in patients undergoing prostate brachytherapy. Urol Oncol 2000; 5:112–117.
23. Brachman DG, Thomas T, Hilbe J, Beyer DC. Failure-free survival following brachytherapy alone or external beam irradiation alone for T1-2 prostate tumors in 2222 patients: results from a single practice. Int J Radiat Oncol Biol Phys 2000; 48:111–117.
24. Ragde H, Korb LJ, Elgamal AA, Grado GL, Nadir BS. Modern prostate brachytherapy. Cancer 2000; 89:135–141.
25. Grimm PD, Blasko JC, Sylvester JE, Meier RM, Cavanagh W. 10-year biochemical (prostate specific antigen) control of prostate cancer with I-125 brachytherapy. Int J Radiat Oncol Biol Phys 2001; 51:31–40.
26. Critz FA, Williams WH, Levinson AK, Benton JB, Holladay CT, Schnell FJ. Simultaneous irradiation for prostate cancer: intermediate results with modern techniques. J Urol 2000; 164:738–734.
27. Lee LN, Stock RG, Stone NN. The role of hormone therapy in the management of intermediate to high risk prostate cancer treated with permanent radioactive seed implantation. Int J Rad Oncol Bio Phys 2002; 52(2):444–452.
28. Stock RG, Cahlon O, Cesaretti J, Kolhmeier MA, Stone NN. Combined modality treatment in the management of high risk prostate cancer. Int J Rad Oncol Biol Phys 2004; 59:1352–1359.
29. Zeitlin SI, Sherman J, Raboy A, Lederman G, Albert, P. High dose combination radiotherapy for the treatment of localized prostate cancer. J Urol 1998; 160:91–94.
30. Gelblum DA, Potters L, Ashley R, Waldbaum R, Wang X-H, Leibel S. Urinary morbidity following ultrasound-guided transperineal prostate seed implantation. Int J Radiat Oncol Biol Phys 1999; 45:59–67.
31. Merrick GS, Butler WM, Lief JH, Dorsey LT. Temporal resolution of urinary morbidity following prostate brachytherapy. Int J Radiat Oncol Biol Phys 2000; 47:121–128.
32. Benoit RM, Naslund M, Cohen JL. Complications after prostate brachytherapy in the medicare population. Urology 2000; 55:91–96.
33. Kleinberg L, Wallner K, Roy J, Zelefsky M, Arterbery VE et al. Treatment-related symptoms during the first year following transperineal ^{125}I prostate implantation. Int J Radiat Oncol Biol Phys 1994; 28:985–990.

34. Desai J, Stock RG, Stone NN, Iannuzzi C, DeWyngaert JK. Acute morbidity following I-125 interstitial implantation of the prostate gland. Radiat Oncol Invest 1998; 6:135–141.
35. Arterbery VE, Wallner K, Roy J, Fuks Z. Short-term morbidity from CT-planned transperineal I-125 prostate implants. Int J Radiat Oncol Biol Phys 1993; 25:661–677.
36. Lee WR, McQuellon RP, Harris-Henderson K, Caase LD, McCullough DL. A preliminary analysis of health-related quality of life in the first year after permanent source interstitial brachytherapy for clinically localized prostate cancer. Int J Radiat Oncol Biol Phys 2000; 46:27.
37. Zelefsky MJ, Wallner KE, Ling CC, Raben A, Hollister T, Wolfe T, Grann A, Gaudin P, Fuks Z, Liebel S. Comparison of 5 year outcome and morbidity of three dimensional conformal radiotherapy versus transperineal permanent iodine-125 implantation for early stage prostatic cancer. J Clin Oncol 1999; 17:517.
38. Brown D, Colonias A, Miller R, Benoit R, Cohen J, Arshoun Y, Galloway M, Karlovits S, Wu A, Johnson M, Quinn A, Kalnicki S. Urinary morbidity with a modified peripheral loading technique of transperineal I-125 implantation. Int J Radiat Oncol Biol Phys 2000; 47:353.
39. Stock RG, Stone NN, Dalal M. Patient reported long term urinary morbidity and quality of life following I-125 prostate brachytherapy. J Urol 2000; 163: 1268a.
40. Ragde H, Blasko JC, Grimm PD, Kenny GM, Sylvester JE et al. Interstitial iodine-125 radiation without adjuvant therapy in the treatment of clinically localized prostate carcinoma. Cancer 1997; 80:442–453.
41. Talcott JA, Clark JA, Stark PC, Mitchell SP. Long-term treatment related complications of brachytherapy for early prostate cancer: a survey of patients previously treated. J Urol 2001; 166:494–499.
42. Stone NN, Ratnow ER, Stock RG. Prior transurethral resection does not increase morbidity following real-time ultrasound guided prostate seed implantation. Tech Urol 2000; 6:123–127.
43. Critz FA, Tarlton RS, Holladay DA. Prostate specific antigen-monitored combination radiotherapy for patients with prostate cancer: I-125 implant followed by external-beam radiation. Cancer 1995; 75:2383–2391.
44. Blasko JC, Wallner K, Grimm PD, Ragde H. PSA based disease control following ultrasound guided I-125 implantation for stage T1/T2 prostatic carcinoma. J Urol 1995; 154:1096–1099.
45. Stock RG, Stone NN, Wesson MF, DeWyngaert JK. A modified technique allowing interactive ultrasound guided three-dimensional transperineal prostate implantation. Int J Radiat Oncol Biol Phys 1995; 32:219–225.
46. Gelbum DY, Potters L. Rectal complications associated with transperineal interstitial brachytherapy for prostate cancer. Int J Radiat Oncol Biol Phys 2000; 48:119–124.
47. Theodorescu D, Gillenwater JY, Schneider BF, Koutrouvelis PG. Prostatourethral–rectal fistula following prostate brachytherapy: incidence and risk factors. J Urol 2000; 163:1294a.
48. Hu K, Wallner K. Clinical course of rectal bleeding following I-125 prostate brachytherapy. Int J Radiat Oncol Biol Phys 1998; 41:263–265.

49. Snyder KM, Stock RG, Hong SM, Lo YC, Stone NN. Defining the risk of developing grade 2 proctitis following I-125 prostate brachytherapy using a rectal dose volume histogram analysis. Int J Rad Oncol Biol Phys 2001; 50:335–341.

50. Potters L, Torre T, Fearn PA, Leibel SA, Kattan MW. Potency after permanent prostate brachytherapy for localized prostate cancer. Int J Radiat Oncol Biol Phys 2001; 50:1235–1242.

51. Stock RG, Kao J, Stone NN. Penile erection function after permanent radioactive seed implantation for treatment of prostate cancer. J Urol 2001; 165:436–439.

3

Transperineal Radiofrequency Interstitial Tumor Ablation of the Prostate

**Bob Djavan, Shirin Milani, Keywan Ghawidel,
and Michael Marberger**

Department of Urology, University of Vienna, Vienna, Austria

Radiofrequency (RF) has been employed to destroy tissue locally in animals as well as in humans. Safety and efficacy of this approach have been demonstrated in the treatment of hepatocellular carcinoma, various metastatic tumors to the liver, osteoid osteomas, and xenografted MXT-tumors in mice (1–4). Rossi et al. (1) concluded that RF interstitial thermal ablation was effective in destroying hepatic tumors within a short treatment time. They showed that the targeted tissue was irreversibly destroyed by coagulative necrosis, with no evidence of venous thrombosis or significant hemorrhage at the border of the lesion. The treatment was performed as an outpatient procedure and the complications observed were minimal (1). RF energy has also been employed extensively to treat benign prostatic hyperplasia with the transurethral needle ablation (TUNA) device. Using a transurethral aproach, coagulative necrosis is produced around the needles inserted into the prostate (5–7).

Transrectal ultrasonography provides real time imaging for accurate needle placement in the prostate. However, the true dimensions of the thermal lesion created cannot be assessed as the sensitivity of the ultrasound image is insufficient to define perfused vs. nonperfused tissues. The lesion size must therefore be predicted accurately at the time of treatment based on physical parameters. In order to monitor treatment efficacy and potential complications, accurate imaging of the lesion is, however, imperative (8).

RF INTERSTITIAL TUMOR ABLATION PROCEDURE

Djavan et al. (9) performed RF interstitial tumor ablation (RITA) in three, four, and three patients with administration of general, spinal, and local anesthesia, respectively, and the patients were then placed in the lithotomy position and prepped as for perineal surgery. A three-way (F 18) Foley catheter was inserted and irrigated with cold saline (15°C) at an infusion rate of 50 cc/min to cool the urethra. The saline solution was cooled prior to treatment only and no cooling was done during treatment. The temperature of the irrigating saline was therefore not maintained. Using a Siemen's Sonoline Versa Ultrasound unit (Erlangen, Germany) with a 7.5 MHz transrectal transducer, measurements of the transverse, anterio-posterior, and cephalo-caudal diameters of the prostate were obtained (9,11).

A 15-gage, three-hook active needle was used to deliver the RF energy. The hooks, when deployed, radiate at an angle of 120° to each other and describe a spheric volume of 2 cm in diameter. Based on this geometry, a $2.0 \times 2.0 \times 2.0$ cm^3 spheric lesion was expected around the active needle. The triple-hook electrodes were also equipped with individual thermocouples mounted on the distal tips of the individual hooks. The distal centimeter of the needle shaft itself was an active electrode as well, as were all of the hooks when deployed from the tip. The remainder of the needle shaft was insulated both thermally and electrically. Each needle electrode had an infusion port in order to modify the impedance of the lesion as needed.

A 50 W monopolar RF generator (Model 500P) operating at a frequency of 460 kHz was used. Patients were grounded by a specially designed grounding pad applied near the hip. The generator offers impedance measurements for the system, measurements of the total amount of energy delivered in joules, and individual readings for each of the various thermocouples mounted on the hooks of the needles. Furthermore, it has a window to read three independent temperature measurements, recorded by independent thermosensistors, mounted on a needle at 5 mm intervals and placed between the prostate and the rectum. The generator is equipped with an RS-232 port for downloading information into a special computer program. The program records real time temperatures and impedance.

All needles were placed under transrectal ultrasound guidance and viewed carefully in both the sagittal and the transverse planes to ensure that they were in the appropriate position as decided in the preoperative treatment plan.

The independent thermocouple was initially placed between the prostate and the rectum, posterior to the lobe of the treated area. The active needle was then placed according to the desired location and measurement, and the treatment was started. A total of 21 lesions were produced in 10 patients. Nine patients had two lesions and one patient had three lesions. All lesions were placed in the lateral lobes of the prostate (one or two on each side). If one of the three prostate diameters was below 4 cm, the capsular region was also included in the treatment zone (9).

An initial power of 10 W was selected and the timer was arbitrarily set to 10 min. The treatment plan was essentially designed to raise the temperature at each individual hook to ∼100°C in 2–3 min and to maintain that temperature for another 3 min. The operator can control and adjust the amount of power needed in order to achieve these goals. When the desired temperatures were reached and maintained for the prescribed period of time, a cool-down period to verify completeness of the lesion was undertaken. During cool down, the power was turned off and the temperature at each hook was observed for 60 s. Based on the experience with RF in treating human tissue, a drop in temperature below 55°C within 60 s predicted an incomplete lesion (1–4). Finally, the hooks were retracted and the needle repositioned for a new lesion.

HISTOPATHOLOGICAL FEATURES

The predictability and reproducibility of the thermal lesion induced with RITA was investigated by Djavan et al. (9) and Zlotta et al. (10). They evaluated the utility of magnetic resonance imaging (MRI) for postoperative treatment monitoring, as well as the clinical efficacy and feasibility of RITA in the treatment of localized prostate cancers (PCa) by analyzing serum prostate-specific antigen (PSA) velocity and biopsy results at 3, 6, and 12 months posttreatment. Patient quality of life and treatment-related complications were also recorded. Ten patients with localized PC, aged 66–74 years (average 71 ± 1.8 years) were included in the study. Average preoperative serum PSA and average Gleason score (GS) were 11.5 ± 2.6 ng/mL (range 7–16) and 5.8 ± 2 (range 3–8), respectively. Patients were scheduled for radical prostatectomy and underwent RITA treatment (RITA Medical Systems, Mountain View, CA) with an endorectal MRI before and 1 day after RITA. The size of the specific lesions was calculated and predicted prior to needle placement according to the geometry of the shaped needle array. Radical retropubic prostatectomy was performed 1–7 days after RITA (11).

A total of 21 single lesions were created. Plateau temperatures of 100°C at the tips of the triple-hook electrode were reached at an average of 140 ± 33 s. The plateau temperature of 100°C was maintained for 180 s. Impedance remained stable at an average of 56 Ω throughout the procedure. In 19 lesions the thermal curve and especially the cool-down phase were adequate (temperature >55°C during cool down). However, in two lesions the temperature at the active electrodes dropped below 55°C after 60 s of cool down. No major increase in temperature was observed with the independent thermocouple inserted between the prostate and the rectum. RITA-induced changes were clearly visible as hypointense foci on T1-weighted, gadolinium-enhanced, spin-echo images. On T2-weighted images, all lesions presented as homogenous areas of high signal intensity. However, demarcation of the lesions was less good compared with the Gd-enhanced images. In total 19 lesions, similar in shape, were observed. In the remaining two lesions, only irregular areas of higher signal intensity were noted. Zonal discrimination was lost and the lesions were mainly located in the upper two-thirds of the prostate. Of the 10 patients, three had capsular penetration on MR images, which was confirmed on pathologic examination. Findings on the dynamic images did not add further infomation to the findings on the delayed, gadolinium-enhanced images. On T1-weighted, gadolinium-enhanced, spin-echo images, lesion volumes ranged from 3.04 to 10.60 cm^3 (volume = $1/6 \times \pi(a \times b \times c)$), where a, b, and c are maximal radii in the transverse, anterio-posterior, and craniocaudal directions, respectively).

At the time of surgery, no major change in the nature and consistency of the prostate was noted. However, some increased vascularity of the gland was observed. Histological mapping of the thermic lesion was possible in all prostate specimens and showed coagulative necrosis. The necrotic portion was consistently found in the posterior and paraurethral parts of the gland surrounding the placement of RF needle electrodes. However, in the same two lesions, which were already irregular on MRI and which had an inadequate cool-down phase, patchy areas of necrosis were noticed, giving the impression of an incomplete lesion. In these two cases, volume measurement was not possible.

The other lesions were located in the lateral lobes of the prostate, extending from the periurethral zone to the capsular region of the specimen. In one case, the posterior and lateral parts of the urethra were involved. In six cases, ejaculatory ducts were within the necrotic area. In patients treated immediately before surgery, necrosis was visible as an indistinct zone of pale tissue. After 24 h the area was evident macroscopically as hemorrhagic necrosis. In 7 of 10 patients, the cancer area was totally or partly within the RITA lesions.

The destroyed area showed sharp boundaries. In fresh lesions epithelial cells exhibited small, dark staining, pycnotic nuclei. The surrounding cytoplasm was narrow and irregularly vacuolated. The epithelium was detached from the basal layer or from basement membrane and the single cells were dissociated from one another. The interstitial connective tissue was edematous and erythrocytes within the blood vessels were sticking together and showed damaged membranes. After 24 h a hemorrhagic necrosis was seen in the prostate. Early organization by granulation tissue could be noticed at 7 days post-RITA.

Average lesion diameters as seen on MRI were 2.08 ± 0.23 cm (transverse diameter) $\times$ 2.09 ± 0.36 cm (anterio-posterior diameter) $\times$ 2.28 ± 0.21 cm (cephalo-caudal). Average lesion diameters at histology were

2.20 $\pm$ 0.23 $\times$ 2.10 $\pm$ 0.31 $\times$ 2.38 $\pm$ 0.14 cm, respectively. Average lesion volume was 5.37 $\pm$ 1.83 cm^3 on MRI vs. 5.86 $\pm$ 1.63 cm^3 in the histopathological specimen. There were no statistically significant differences when comparing both groups ($p = 0.377$). No side effects were seen. No patient experienced rectal discomfort, internal hemorrhage, or external hemorrhage.

Specifically, postoperative MRI revealed no alterations of the rectum, neurovascular bundle, or the region of the external urethral sphincter.

POST-RITA PSA VELOCITY

In a second study (11), 20 patients with clinical localized PC (T1–2), aged 66–74 years (average 71 $\pm$ 1.8 years) underwent RITA with a curative attempt. The average preoperative serum PSA and average GS were 11.5 $\pm$ 2.6 ng/mL (range 7–16) and 5.8 $\pm$ 2 (range 3–10), respectively.

An average of 10 single lesions were created per patient. Plateau temperatures of 100°C at the tips of the triple-hook electrode were reached at an average of 140 $\pm$ 33 s. The plateau temperature of 100°C was maintained for 180 s. Impedance remained stable at an average of 56 Ω throughout the procedure. No major increase in temperature was observed with the independent thermocouple inserted between the prostate and the rectum. Mean hospital stay was 1.8 days (range 1–4). Mean patient age, serum PSA, and GS were 71.4 years (range 66–75), 10.5 $\pm$ 3 ng/mL (range 3–19), and 5.8 $\pm$ 2 (range 3–9), respectively. The stage distribution was as follows: T1 ($n = 2$), T2 ($n = 21$), T3 ($n = 7$).

Mean follow-up was 12 months (range 10–24). After an initial increase at 2 weeks to a mean of 36.4 $\pm$ 8 ng/mL, the PSA level dropped to 1.1 ng/mL (range 0.01–3.8) at 12 weeks. The positive biopsy rate at 12 weeks was 30.7% (4/13), all of which had a GS of >7 or a pre-RITA PSA level >15 ng/mL. At 12 months biopsy results were available on 29 patients. Residual cancer was found in 13/29 (44%) patients following RITA, while 16/29 (55%) had no evidence of persistent cancer tissue. In addition, significant improvements in maximal flow rate (Q_{max}), international prostate symptom score (IPSS), and quality of life were noted. Initial hematuria and erectile dysfunction were noted in 12/30 (40%) and 2/30 (6.6%) patients, respectively. Prostatic obstruction requiring transurethral resection of the prostate was noted in one patient and transient incontinence (>3 pads/day) in 2/30 (6.6%) patients (10).

Minimally invasive treatment modalities for PCa treatment such as cryosurgery (12–14) and high-intensity focused ultrasound (15) have recently seen renewed interest because of promising clinical reports, low morbidity, minimal blood loss, and short hospital stay. Previously, RF energy was delivered via a transurethral route for the treatment of benign prostatic hyperplasia (BPH) (5–7). However, in contrast to BPH, the therapy of PCa requires destruction of the entire organ, as PCa is frequently located in the peripheral zone and is by nature a multifocal disease. RITA was therefore performed through a transperineal approach, using higher power as for BPH. This approach is shared by other minimal invasive treatment modalities of localized PCa such as brachytherapy and cryosurgery for similar reasons (14,16).

Although cryoablation of the prostate creates a hypoechoic zone with a hyperechoic rim (ice ball), the size of the lesion does not correlate with the extent of tissue destruction. With RITA, the changes seen at ultrasonography are transient in nature and appear as "speckled" hyperechoic snow flakes that, within 20 min of the procedure, begin to dissipate. These changes are most likely due to the generation of vapor created by the boiling of intra- and extra-cellular water as the temperature reaches 100°C. They likewise, however, do not correlate with the zone of actual coagulative necrosis obtained. The resolution and discrimination of currently available ultrasonography equipment is insufficient to distinguish viable from necrotic tissues. RF ablation with the RITA technique destroys the gland simultaneously by direct heating from the electrode and by conduction. RF produces ionic or molecular agitation and a collision of particles in accordance with the frequency of the energy wave generated. This produces heat in a very localized area around the point source, resulting in a central hot core. The continued delivery of RF energy supports the central core of heat, which then distributes this heat by conduction to the surrounding tissue to produce the final lesion. The size of the lesion is a function of the thermal properties of the tissue and the time during which the "hot core" is maintained. Thus, the dimensions of the thermal lesion created by RF energy can be predicted and planned according to tissue impedance, power delivery, time of application, and total energy delivered to the tissue (17).

The initial setting of 10 W is based on the mean impedance monitored by the electrode and measured by the generator. Impedance is a crucial factor in the size and evolution of the thermal lesion. It reflects the degree of tissue hydration and the ability to transfer heat. As it is also a function of the surface area of the electrode monitoring the impedance, it is a relative number, which is low with a large surface area of the electrode and high when the surface is small. Tissue displaying high impedance values therefore requires less power and time for ablation, but tends to produce smaller lesions. The needle electrodes employed in RITA therapy are engineered so that the relative impedance of the prostate is at a convenient level to produce the desired lesions in a short period of time. Size and configuration of the electrodes also determine the shape of the lesion. Provided the needles are placed correctly, RF energy creates predictable and reproducible lesions.

Analysis of MRI imaging and histological examination revealed good correlation and no statistically significant difference in volume and size of the lesion. On the basis of these data, it was concluded that lesion size is accurately verifiable on MRI (9,11).

TREATMENT MONITORING

The cool-down cycle is crucial as a method of treatment assessment and control. The cool-down cycle is a measurement of the fall in temperature of the lesion in terms of dissipation of heat. Heat is dissipated, regardless of the source, by conduction and convection. Conduction is the heating and cooling of adjacent cells or tissue as one goes farther from the heat source. As such, there is an obvious, measurable decrease in tissue temperature as the distance $(1/r^4)$ increases. A fall in temperature below 55°C indicates an incomplete thermal lesion. In a perfect model there is a smooth, gradual decreasing temperature gradient, indicating a "sealed lesion". If at some point prior to arriving at the borders of the lesion, a rapid drop in temperature occurs, then this would no longer represent "conductive losses" but rather a convective loss, that is, persisting vascularized tissue. This rapid drop in temperature basically represents viable, perfused tissue. Based on these phenomena, the cool-down cycle, rather than the ultrasonographic imaging, is the essential intraoperative feedback to verify the completeness of treatment.

In two lesions where the temperature fell below 55°C within 60 s of cool down, these areas were not re-treated in order to obtain correlation with MRI and histology (11). In fact, MRI and histology were not able to detect a complete lesion and showed viable tissue between small necrotic areas of irregular shape. As a consequence, if the temperature falls below 55°C during the cool down, the same area must be retreated.

Because the wavelength of RF energy is far too long to create distant, unwanted damage, significant side effects on adjacent organs were not expected and this was confirmed. In addition, RF-induced lesions were shown to be predictable in size and location. The procedure was easy to perform under spinal and even local anesthesia. Regarding the clinical efficacy, it is obvious that a larger number of patients and a longer follow-up is required to make a final judgement. After an initial increase at 2 weeks to a mean of 36.4 + 8 ng/mL, PSA dropped to 1.1 ng/mL (range 0.01–3.8) at 12 weeks. Positive biopsy rate at 12 weeks was 20% (4/20), all of which had a GS > 7 or a pre-RITA PSA >15 ng/mL. These data indicate significant ablation of prostatic tissue and warrant further investigation. The combination of the current technology with a three-dimensional ultrasound guided insertion technique may further improve clinical efficacy and reduce eventual complications.

FUTURE CONCEPTS WITH RITA

Recently, a novel technique has been developed using electrolyte solutions infused through the RF electrode (22-gage hollow stainless-steel needle) into the prostatic tissue, thus creating a so called "virtual electrode" (18–20). Hypertonic saline solutions (14.6%) can have up to 25 times better conductivity than blood or body fluids such as lymph, urine, or semen and 60–75 times better than many tissues (i.e., prostate tissue). Interstitial electrolyte perfusion spreads RF current further into the tissue, away from the surface of the electrode, thus allowing a greater amount of RF energy to be delivered to the tissue without reaching the critical current density and avoiding desiccation and char formation at the electrode–tissue interface. Therefore, tissue impedance can be controlled and lesion size augmented. Variation of concentration and volume of electrolyte solution delivered allows one to achieve larger lesion sizes in shorter times (seconds). In addition, thermocouples can be embedded on the needle shaft to ensure accurate temperature monitoring during RF delivery.

Undoubtedly, as should be required for any minimally invasive treatment device, lesion size should be controllable and predictable with respect to size, shape, and location within the prostate gland. The lesion should be complete and no areas should be spared from coagulation necrosis within the lesion. These requirements were evaluated by Hoey et al. (18,20) as well as Leveillee et al. (19). Tissue effects were determined in five mongrel dogs in a chronic study (0.5–8 weeks). All animals recovered uneventfully and were later sacrificed. Macroscopically, lesion shape was regular and reproducible. Histologically, coagulation necrosis was observed in 69.9% ± 16% of the glands treated. Lesion size was limited only by the duration of RF energy application (19). Hoey and Co-workers, compared conventional RF treatment to RF treatment using this new virtual saline-liquid electrode in a series of 10 dogs. Mean lesion size was 0.34 cc (range 0.06–0.93 cc) and 8.54 cc (range 2.53–22.88 cc) for the conventional and virtual electrodes, respectively, suggesting that the saline-liquid electrode allowed creation of significantly larger lesions than the conventional electrode. Time to increase of impedance was significantly shorter with the conventional electrode, suggesting that tissue desiccation, which would subsequently limit lesion size, occurred much earlier than with the saline-liquid electrode (20). Although the TUNA system employs the conventional electrode, the system self-regulates the wattage output based on tissue temperature and impedance feedback to avoid tissue evaporation and charring.

Recently, Djavan and Hoey (21) evaluated the feasibility of transurethral prostate ablation using the saline-liquid electrode introduced via a flexible cystoscope in dogs. The instrument was introduced into the urethra via a small perineal urethrostomy incision (due to the U-shape of the canine urethra and the penile bone in dogs). The electrode could be inserted into the lobes bilaterally without complication. Obviously, the capability of varying lesion size is crucial and essential when various gland volumes are to be treated. In the same study, the authors delivered RF energy with the saline-liquid electrode for 30, 45, 60, and 90 s and correlated their findings with the histopathological specimens. Average lesion volumes were 1.76 cc at 30 s, 2.42 cc at 45 s, 3.96 cc at 60 s, and 5.03 cc at 90 s. Thus, energy delivery time allows prediction of lesion size in the prostate with this new technique (21,22).

These findings were to be expected since the electrical conductivity of the tissue is determined primarily by the saline concentration field and is therefore a function of time and space. Since the saline infusion is maintained over time, a saline concentration field with high conductivity develops, creating a virtual saline-liquid electrode, where lesion size and shape can be controlled by changing the length of the active electrode in the prostate as well as by varying RF energy delivery time.

In a recent canine study, thermal mapping of RFT lesions in the prostate was presented (23). Thermal measurements were recorded at known tissue depths radiating outward from the active electrode. This study confirmed the rapid heating of tissue using the wet-electrode and RFT system with temperatures reaching 100°C near the active electrode. Lesion size measured correlated with the thermal map. The preliminary, interim data confirm the ability of this technology to rapidly ablate animal and human prostate tissue using an endoscopic approach and suggest clinical safety with reasonable effectiveness.

CONCLUSIONS

Transperineal RITA is able to create predictable and reproducible lesions in the human prostate. Endorectal MRI was able to visualize and verify the dimensions of the thermal lesion found on histopathology. The procedure was safe and no major side effects were noted. RITA was performed under spinal but also under local anesthesia and was well tolerated. In this early clinical phase, PSA dropped significantly at 12 weeks post-RITA. Persistently elevated PSA (>0.5 ng/mL) and positive biopsies were always related to patients with high risk of systemic disease (GS >7 and PSA >15 ng/mL). Nevertheless, with the current technology and needle designs, areas of viable tissue were frequently observed on histopathology, although these respective areas were primarily aimed to be treated. Despite advantages related to low costs, easy handling, safety, and feasibility of the procedure, RITA is still to be considered an investigational tool, requiring improvements specifically in the energy delivery device.

REFERENCES

1. Rossi S, Di Stasi M, Buscarini E, Cavanna L, Quaretti P, Squassante E, Garbagnati F, Buscarini L. Percutaneous radiofrequency interstitial thermal ablation in the treatment of small hepatocellular carcinoma. Cancer J Sci Am 1995; 1:73–81.
2. De Berg JC, Pattynama PMT, Obermaun WRI, Bode PJ, Vielvoyr GJ, Taminiau AHM. Percutaneous computed-tomography-guided thermocoagulation for osteoid osteomas. Lancet 1995; 346:350–351.
3. Zlotta AR, Kiss R, De Decker R, Schulman CC. MXT mammary tumor treatment with a high temperature radiofrequency ablation device. Int J Oncol 1995; 7:863–869.
4. Calkins H, Langberg J, Sousa J, El-Atassi R, Leon A, Kou W, Kalbfleisch S, Morady F. Radiofrequency catheter ablation of assessory atrioventricular connections in 250 patients. Circulation 1992; 85:1337–1346.
5. Schulman CC, Zlotta AR, Rasor J, Hourriez L, Noel JC, Edwards SD. Transurethral needle ablation (TUNA): safety, feasibility, and tolerance of a new office procedure for treatment of benign prostatic hyperplasia. Eur Urol 1993; 24:415–423.
6. Schulman CC, Zlotta AR. Transurethral needle ablation of the prostate for treatment of benign prostatic hyperplasia: early clinical experience. Urology 1995; 45:28–33.
7. Oesterling JE, Issa MM, Roehrborn CG, Bruskewitz R, Naslund MJ, Perez-Marrero R, Shumaker BP. Long-term results of a prospective, randomized clinical trial comparing TUNA® to TURP for the treatment of symptomatic BPH. J Urol 1997; 157:A328.

8. Parivar F, Hricak H, Shinohara K, Kurhanewicz J, Vigneron DB, Nelson SJ, Carroll PR. Detection of locally recurrent prostate cancer after cryosurgery: evaluation by transrectal ultrasound, magnetic resonance imaging, and three-dimensional proton magnetic resonance spectroscopy. Urology 1996; 48:594–599.
9. Djavan B, Susani M, Shariat S, Zlotta AR, Silverman DE, Schulman CC, Marberger M. Transperineal radiofrequency interstitial tumor ablation (RITA) of the prostate. Tech Urol 1998; 4(2):103–109.
10. Zlotta AR, Djavan B, Matos C, Noel JC, Peny MO, Silverman DE, Marberger M, Schulmann CC. Percutaneus transperineal radiofrequency ablation of prostate tumor: safety, feasibility and pathological effects on human prostate cancer. Br J Urol 1998; 81(2):265–275.
11. Djavan B, Zlotta AR, Susani M, Heinz G, Shariat S, Silverman DE, Schulman CC, Marberger M. Transperineal radiofrequency interstitial tumor ablation of the prostate: correlation of magnetic resonance imaging with histopathologic examination. Urology 1997; 50(6):986–993.
12. Cox RL, and Crawford ED. Complicatons of cryosurgical ablation of the prostate to treat localized adenocarcinoma of the prostate. Urology 1995; 45:932–935.
13. Grampsas SA, Miller GJ, Crawford ED. Salvage radical prostatectomy after failed transperineal cryotherapy; histologic findings from prostate whole-mount specimens correlated with intraoperative transrectal ultrasound images. Urology 1995; 45:936–941.
14. Blasko JC, Ragde H, Luse RW, Sylvester JE, Cavanagh W, Grimm PD. Should brachytherapy be considered a therapeutic option in localized prostate cancer. Urol Clin North Am 1996; 23:633–650.
15. Madersbacher S, Pedevilla M, Vingers L, Susani M, Marberger M. Effect of high-intensity focused ultrasound on human prostate cancer in vivo. Cancer Res 1995; 55:3346–3351.
16. Wieder J, Schmidt JD, Casola G, van Sonnenberg E, Stainken BF, Parsons CL. Transrectal ultrasound-guided transperineal cryoablation in the treatment of prostate carcinoma: preliminary results. J Urol 1995; 154:435–441.
17. Organ LW. Electophysiologic principles of radiofrequency lesion making. Appl Neurphysiol 1976; 39:69–76.
18. Hoey MF, Leveille RJ, Hulbert JC et al. A new method to couple radiofrequency energy to prostate tissue using electrolyte solution to enhance ablation. J Endourol 1995; 9:A125.
19. Leveillee RJ, Hoey MF, Hulbert JC et al. Enhanced radiofrequency ablation of canine prostate utilizing a liquid conductor: the virtual electrode. J Endourol 1996; 10:5–11.
20. Hoey MF, Mulier P, Levellee RJ et al. Transurethral prostate ablation with saline electrode allows controlled production of larger lesions than conventional methods. J Endourol 1997; 11:279–284.
21. Hoey MF, Dixon CM, Paul S. Transurethral prostate ablation using saline liquide electrode introduced via flexible cystoscope. J Endourol 1998; 12:461–468.
22. Djavan B, Hoey MF, Dixon CM et al. Transurethral tissue ablation of the canine prostate with radiofrequency energy using a novel saline electrode. Eur Urol 1998; 33:A74.
23. Hoey MF, Dixon CM, Hong E et al. Correlation of interstitial temperature measurement to developed lesion size in the prostate using radiofrequency at the liquid electrode. J Urol 1999; 161:A4.

4

Laparoscopic Radical Prostatectomy

**Clément-Claude Abbou, András Hoznek,
David B. Samadi, Safwat K. Zaki, Leif E. Olsson,
and Laurent Salomon**

*Service d'Urologie, Centre Hospitalier Universitaire Henri Mondor,
Créteil, France*

Laparoscopy has become an integral part of urologic surgery. Its indications have been progressively extended to the most advanced oncologic and reconstructive procedures. Within this frame, radical prostatectomy is of major interest considering the incidence and clinical significance of prostate cancer. The procedure comprises several steps of challenging dissection where the preservation of delicate nerve and muscular structures should be conciliated with safe tumor excision. The intervention ends with vesicourethral anastomosis, which is considered the most difficult reconstructive procedure in urologic laparoscopy.

Laparoscopic radical prostatectomy has become gradually a wholly standardized procedure and it is now routinely performed in several centers throughout the world. We describe in this chapter a series of steps, which involves performing this procedure safely and accurately.

SURGICAL TECHNIQUE

We describe our operative technique based on our experience with more than 250 procedures.

Patient Selection, Preoperative Preparation

The body habitus of the patient has usually not significantly influenced the degree of difficulty of the surgery. However, in obese patients access creation may be more difficult. The thickness of the abdominal wall diminishes the available length of the trocars and consequently the ability to reach deeply situated structures with the instruments. Obese patients frequently have a large amount of peri-vesical fat and the bladder may be difficult to retract during the vesicourethral anastomosis. It often obstructs the view on the bladder neck and urethra when using a 0° laparoscope. The 30° laparoscope may be a valuable help in these circumstances.

Previous abdominal surgery sometimes leads to parietal or intestinal adhesions, which may increase risks during access creation.

Periprostatic fibrosis increases the difficulty of dissecting the prostate, particularly on its posterior aspect. This situation is often met after neoadjuvant hormone therapy, previous prostatitis, repeated transrectal biopsies, previous transurethral resection of the prostate (TURP), or retropubic prostatectomy.

Patients should remain on low residue diet for 3–4 days before surgery; this facilitates the retraction of the bowels during the surgical resection.

Patient Positioning, Access Creation

Since the intervention lasts for several hours under general anesthesia, the positioning of the patient should be done very meticulously to avoid decubitus lesions or neuromuscular injury. The patient is placed supine in steep Trendelenburg position. Spreader bars enable the legs to be opened 30°. Silicon pads are used in order to protect pressure points. We do not use shoulder holders, which involve the risk of nerve compression.

After prepping the skin from the xyphoid process to midthigh, drapes are placed in a sterile fashion and an 18-French three-way catheter is inserted into the bladder.

We use five trocars. First, we perform a hemi-circumferential incision at the lower margin of the umbilicus. Open Hasson technique is used to gain access to the abdominal cavity under direct vision. Other sites of primary access can be used in the presence of surgical scar around the umbilicus. Then, a 12 mm trocar with a foam grip is inserted, the abdomen is insufflated. The abdominal cavity is inspected thoroughly. The Trendelenburg position is exaggerated to 30°, which displaces the bowels, cephalad by gravity. In case of adhesions, an intact site is chosen for the first trocar puncture. Throughout the whole procedure, the insufflation pressure is maintained below 10–12 mmHg. However, during puncture with secondary trocars, it is safer to increase CO_2 pressure to 20 mmHg. This prevents the abdominal wall from coming in close contact with the bowels and vascular structures, thus diminishing the risk of trocar injury. In the presence of parietal bowel adhesions, they can be easily detached with monopolar rotating-tip coagulating scissors before the insertion of all other trocars. The monopolar scissors should be used very carefully because they can cause thermal injury to the bowels. During laparoscopy, we use both monopolar and bipolar electrocautery. The advantage of monopolar scissors is that they can resect and coagulate at the same time. In contrast, the bipolar electrocautery can only be used for hemostatasis. The monopolar is handled by the primary surgeon and the assistant is responsible for activating the bipolar.

Several factors should be taken into account when choosing the site of the trocars. Trocars should be sufficiently distanced from each other to prevent collisions between instruments and to offer an optimal angle between instruments during the step of suturing. Given the limited length of the instruments, there is a limit above which trocars cannot be placed; otherwise instruments would not reach structures below the pubic symphysis. With these considerations in mind, we elaborated a five-trocar configuration (Fig. 4.1).

The use of large trocars is another source of complications. Postoperative hernias occur only at the level of 10 or 12 mm trocars. Therefore, the number of large trocars should be limited to a minimum. In our practice, we use only two 12 mm trocars: one for the laparoscope and a second one near the lateral margin of the rectus sheath on the surgeon's side. The latter is indispensable for bringing down the needles and large instruments like vascular clip appliers. Parietal bleedings rarely occur during trocar insertion. The typical site is at the two trocars near the lateral margin of the rectus sheath. These bleedings are due to injury of the branches of the inferior epigastric artery. This incident can be managed with the use of a balloon trocar that compresses the vessels. The drawback is the impossibility of pushing this trocar deep into the abdomen,

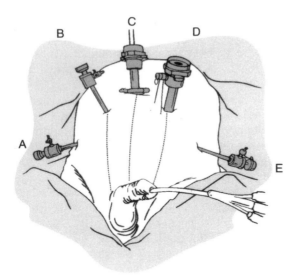

Figure 4.1   The five-trocar configuration.

thus reducing the available length of the instruments. However, this method is usually satisfactory; at the end of the procedure each trocar is removed under direct vision to insure no residual bleeding.

Posterior Dissection

The pouch of Douglas is widely exposed. Insufflation pressure is diminished to 12 mmHg. In order to get a better visualization of the pouch, it is helpful to retract the sigmoid colon cephalad and to the left of the abdominal wall using a straight transcutaneous needle. This is passed under vision through an appendix epiploicae and then again through the abdominal wall. The sigmoid is lifted with the suture and fixed with a straight clamp.

The peritoneum is incised over the vasa deferentia and the seminal vesicles. The vas deferens is usually easily identified, because it deforms the surface of the overlying peritoneum. There is, however, a risk of confusing it with the ureter and therefore, the laparoscopic anatomy of these two structures must be well understood. When inspecting the anterior aspect of the Douglas pouch, two transverse inverted U-shaped peritoneal folds can be observed. The more superficial fold corresponds to the ureters and the deeper to the distal portion of the vasa deferentia. The transverse peritoneotomy should be done on this deeper fold. The dissection continues along the posterior surface of the seminal vesicles downward, and Denonvilliers' fascia is incised. It is important not to dissect the vasa and seminal vesicles free of the bladder base at this step, otherwise these structures will hang and obstruct the view when dealing with the prostato-rectal cleavage.

The latter is performed at both sides of the rectum until the levator ani muscles are reached. The vasa deferentia are dissected and sectioned only when this is done (Fig. 4.2). During the dissection of the seminal vesicles, it should be remembered that the cavernous nerves are in close relationship with the tip of the seminal vesicles. Two large arteries are typically identified supplying each seminal vesicle from the lateral side. These are divided immediately adjacent to the seminal vesicles after being controlled with surgical clips. When nerve sparing is included in the goals of the surgery, we prefer to use hemoclips rather than any kind of thermal energy to achieve hemostasis of these vessels. The vas deferentia are clipped and divided. Anterior attachments to these structures are dissected using blunt and monopolar scissors dissection until the location of the bladder neck.

Again, previous TURP, multiple biopsies, prostatitis, and neoadjuvant hormonal therapy are the main causes that may be responsible of bothersome fibrosis during this dissection.

Dissection of Retzius Space

The dissection of the bladder is much facilitated if it is previously filled with 200 cc of saline, which results in a slight downward traction due to gravity. The upper limit of the bladder in men is particularly high; the incision of the anterior parietal peritoneum should be performed as close to the umbilicus as possible in the midline. The optic is retracted until the two umbilical arteries

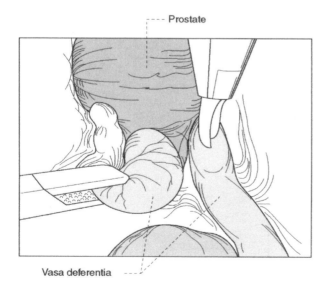

Figure 4.2   Dissected and sectioned vasa deferentia.

and urachus can be identified. There is an avascular plane between the bladder and the abdominal wall. If bleeding occurs, it means that one is too close to the bladder. The peritoneum should be incised laterally, to facilitate the passage of instruments to the deep part of the pelvis. The symphysis pubis is rapidly reached; care should be taken not to injure the small vessels that run perpendicularly to the rami of the pubic bone. These are collaterals between the external iliac vein and the obturator vein (accessory obturator vein). Their bleeding is difficult to stop; however, if it occurs, the bipolar forceps represent the most effective remedy.

The endopelvic fascia is incised on either side of the prostate and incisions carried toward the apex. Bluntly, the levator muscle attachments are peeled off the prostate. The puboprostatic ligaments are divided sharply for a few millimeters to aid in the apical dissection.

Ligature of the Dorsal Venous Complex

The margin between the urethra and dorsal vein complex is easily identified due to the superb light conditions and magnification of the laparoscope (Fig. 4.3). A 2-0 Vicryl stitch is introduced and secured around the superficial tissue at the base of the prostate and a long tail is left to be used for retraction. The assistant grasps the stitch and retracts posteriorly to put stretch on the apex. A second 2-0 Vicryl stitch is used to place a figure of eight stitch around the Santorini plexus. We prefer intracorporal knotting. It is more precise than extracorporal knotting,

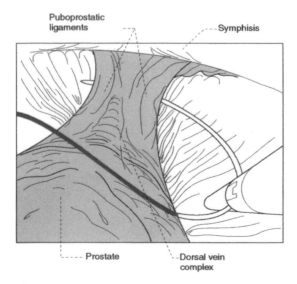

Figure 4.3 The margin between the urethra and dorsal vein complex.

because the knot can be brought farther under the symphysis. The dorsal vein complex is not divided at this step.

Transection of the Bladder Neck

We begin the transection at the anterior aspect of the bladder neck, a few millimeters cephalad to the distal suture of the dorsal venous complex. Because of the lack of manual palpation, the identification of the bladder neck differs from open surgery. The recognition of the landmarks is facilitated by a couple of rules (Fig. 4.4). The consistency of the prostate and that of the bladder are totally different. The prostate is a solid gland, whereas the bladder is mobile when palpating with endoscopic instruments. In addition, the prostate is covered laterally by a plain fascial layer, while the bladder is surrounded by fatty tissue.

To facilitate the transection of the bladder neck, the assistant retracts anteriorly on the prostate base stitch to elevate the bladder neck. The section is carried out between the muscular fibers of the detrusor and the prostatic capsule. Sharply, the anterior bladder neck is opened, the catheter balloon deflated, and the catheter delivered through the opening. The assistant now grasps the catheter with a toothed grasper. The catheter is pulled at the urethral meatus and is secured with a Kelly clamp, allowing the assistant to elevate the bladder neck with anterior traction. The posterior bladder neck is incised, as well as Denonvilliers' fascia. The surgeon soon encounters an empty space indicating that the primary posterior dissection has been reached. The seminal vesicles and vasa defentia are apparent and delivered anteriorly through the empty space.

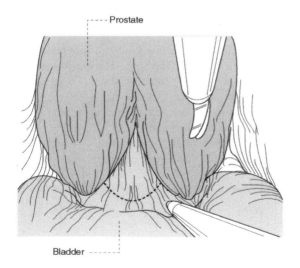

Figure 4.4 Transection of the bladder neck.

The assistant now grasps the left seminal vesicle and retracts toward the right while the suction tip is placed behind the prostate and retracted posteriorly putting the left prostatic pedicle on stretch. The surgeon is able to view the prostate laterally and posteriorly and must progress slowly with clips and sharp dissection until the postero-lateral aspect of the prostate is reached.

When the prostate is not significantly enlarged, the conservation of the bladder neck is facilitated by the enhanced visibility of laparoscopy. However, during the transection of the bladder neck, there are two special circumstances one should be aware of.

The first one occurs after previous TURP. In this situation, the landmarks are blurred and the dissection is rendered more difficult because of periprostatic fibrosis. Special care should be taken when incising the posterior margin of the bladder neck, because of the proximity of the ureters. At the beginning of laparoscopic experience, the distance of the incision line from the ureteral orifices tends to be overestimated due to the magnified vision and the incision may occur too close to the orifices. This leads to two kind of hazardous situations during the step of vesicourethral anastomosis. If the suture is placed too superficially, there is a risk of a tear, resulting in anastomotic leakage. On the other hand, if the suture is placed too deep, it can result in ureteral occlusion. The best way to avoid this situation is to place bilateral double-J stents preoperatively.

The second difficulty is met in the presence of an enlarged median lobe. In this case, the section of the posterior margin of the bladder neck should begin with a submucosal incision, tangentially to the bladder trigone, contouring the bulging median lobe. The danger during this maneuver is to enter the cleavage plane of benign prostatic hyperplasia (BPH), that is, below the surgical capsule of the prostate thus obtaining positive margins.

Apical Dissection

Next, the assistant releases the seminal vesicle and again grasps the proximal stitch on the prostate retracting posteriorly to help expose the apex. The dorsal venous complex is transected between the two previously placed ligatures. This section of the dorsal vein is perpendicular to its axis, but then the plane between the vein and the urethra is developed in an oblique manner caudally. This is important to avoid positive apical margins. Occasionally, the dorsal venous complex gives collaterals to the lateral aspect of the prostate that may bleed. The bipolar forceps permit the achievement of hemostasis. If a nerve sparing is decided, the neurovascular bundles are freed on each side of the urethra (Figs. 4.5 and 4.6). The bundles give perpendicular vascular branches toward the prostate. To avoid thermal injury, we prefer to use hemoclips before sectioning these vessels.

Section of the Lateral Pedicles

The periprostatic fascia has two layers: the outer layer called levator fascia and an inner layer called prostatic fascia. The neurovascular bundles run between these

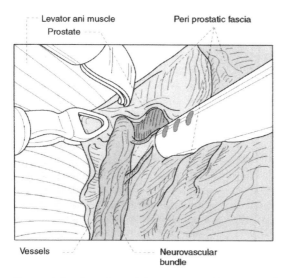

Figure 4.5 One view of the neurovascular bundles freed from the urethra.

two layers. At this point they are in proximity with Dennonvilliers' fascia. If a nerve sparing is decided, the two layers of the periprostatic fascia should be separated and the obturator fascia detached until a subtle groove appears at the lateral aspect of the prostate, indicating the border of the bundles. The bundles can thus

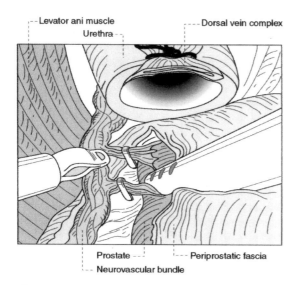

Figure 4.6 Another view of Fig. 4.5.

be detached from the prostate. The assistant grasps the left seminal vesicle and retracts toward the right putting the left prostatic pedicle on stretch. Once the pedicle has been divided in contact with the prostate, the surgeon incises the periprostatic fascia and extends this incision to the apex. The neurovascular bundle is identified and allowed to fall lateral from the prostate by clipping and dividing small branches reaching the prostate as encountered. The right side pedicle and proximal neurovascular bundle preservation are performed in a similar fashion.

During this maneuver, care should be taken not to overstretch the nerves; an elongation of 10% can lead to nerve damage. Again, we use hemoclips before sectioning the vascular branches running toward the prostate. The separation of the bundles is complete when the perirectal fatty tissue appears medially.

Then, the urethra is divided anteriorly and the catheter withdrawn until the posterior urethral mucosa is seen, which is then sharply divided. The assistant, grasping the proximal prostate stitch retracts to each side in an exaggerated manner, allowing the suction tip to be positioned under the rectourethralis and above the rectum permitting the surgeon to complete the prostatectomy. A watertight endocatch is introduced and the prostate placed within. The specimen sac is placed in the upper abdomen.

Vesicourethral Reconstruction

A tennis racket reconstruction is necessary if bladder neck preservation is not possible. This occurs in patients with large BPH, median lobe, or previous TURP. Similarly, if the bladder neck cannot be brought down to the urethra without tension, the solution is to incise sagitally the anterior aspect of the bladder and perform a tennis racket closure posteriorly.

We routinely perform two hemi-circumferential (1) and, more recently, a single circumferential running suture for the anastomosis. The use of a 5/8 tapered needle facilitates the passage of the suture. It is more comfortable to use two needle holders. The right-hand needle holder is inserted through the right paramedian port and the left needle holder through the left lateral port. By doing so, the angle between the needle holders is close to 90°. As a rule of thumb, the right needle holder, which is more vertical, is easier to use at the lateral aspect of the urethra, while the more horizontal left needle holder is used at the top and the bottom of the urethra. A starting knot is performed at the 3 o'clock position in an outside-in fashion, forehand, with the right needle holder on the bladder neck, and inside-out on the urethra. The short tail of the suture is not cut; it will serve to knot the running suture when it is completed. In order to avoid loosing the short tail in the operative field, we attach it with a clip on the anterior aspect of the bladder until the end of the running suture. When the starting knot is done, the needle is passed forehand with the right needle holder from outside-in at the posterior margin of the bladder neck at the 5 o'clock position. The posterior half of the running suture consists of

4–5 needle passages inside-out on the urethra and outside-in on the bladder. The sutures of the urethra are performed forehand, inside-out, with the right needle holder, while the sutures on the bladder are done outside-in, forehand, with the left needle holder (Fig. 4.7). Meanwhile, the assistant helps to retract the bladder neck cranially with the suction-irrigation passed through the left para-median port. In obese patients, it may be difficult to obtain an optimal view of the urethra and bladder neck because of the excessive amount of peri-vesical fat which obstructs the view of the laparoscope. In such cases, it is better to use the 30° laparoscope directed downward. When the posterior half of the running suture is done, the Foley catheter is inserted into the bladder. To perform the anterior half of the running suture, the direction of the needle passage is reversed, at the 9 o'clock position. This is achieved by passing the suture outside-in and then inside-out on the bladder. Then, the suturing goes on outside-in on the urethra and inside-out on the bladder.

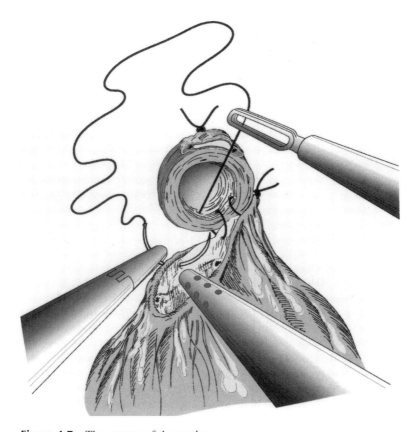

Figure 4.7 The sutures of the urethra

Before inflating the balloon of the Foley catheter, it should be made sure that it was not included in the running suture. The bladder is then filled with 200 cc saline in order to verify the watertightness of the anastomosis.

Specimen Extraction and Closure

The specimen is extracted through the slightly enlarged umbilical port site. There is no direct contact between the surgical specimen and the abdominal wall, because of the use of the watertight endoscopic bag. A small suction drain is inserted through the left lateral 5 mm port site and placed in the Retzius space near the anastomosis.

POSTOPERATIVE CARE

The suction drain can be removed when the amount of evacuated liquid is <50 cc. In the typical patient this occurs on the first postoperative day. If this is not the case and a significant quantity of drainage fluid is observed, a creatinine level determination should be performed. If this analysis reveals lymphorrhea and not urine leakage, the drain should be removed because the lymph is re-absorbed on the peritoneal surface.

At postoperative days 2–4 (day 3 or 4 when done over the weekend) a gravitational cystography is performed in all patients. The bladder is filled with 250 mL of water-soluble contrast, the balloon of the catheter is deflated, and the patient is asked to perform a Valsalva maneuver. With contrast still running, the catheter is slowly pulled and the anastomotic area carefully imaged during Valsalva as well.

When no anastomotic leak is identified, the catheter is immediately removed. If a leak is observed, the catheter should be left in place and another cystography performed 6 days later.

COMPLICATIONS

During open surgery, the main offense to the patient is due to the large incision. In contrast, after laparoscopic radical prostatectomy the typical patient ambulates within the first 48 h and resumes normal activity much faster. If this is not the case a thorough postoperative evaluation should be performed.

Since laparoscopic radical prostatectomy uses a transperitoneal approach in contrast to traditional retropubic prostatectomy, unusual complications may occur.

Rectal injuries may occur during the initial recto-prostatic dissection, or more frequently during the division of the lateral pedicles or the apex of the prostate. Most of the time, these injuries are minimal; they are immediately recognized and repaired, thus avoiding the necessity of temporary colostomy.

Since the peritoneal cavity is opened, postoperative paralytic ileus and abdominal pain are encountered in the patient, with more pronounced intraoperative bleeding or postoperative urine leak due to the irritating effect of blood or urine at the peritoneal surface. These complications usually spontaneously resolve within a few days. As it has been already mentioned, the ureters are at risk of injury during the posterior dissection if they are mistaken for the vas deferens or during the section of the posterior bladder neck, especially in patients with previous TURP. The accurate identification of the anatomic landmarks and the insertion of two double-J stents represent a guarantee to avoid these problems.

Urinary leakage does not have a significant impact on the postoperative course, provided it is recognized in time. Therefore, we routinely perform a retrograde urethrocystogram before taking out the urinary catheter. If a leakage occurs, the catheter should be kept in place for a few more days.

TECHNICAL VARIANTS

Our operative technique described earlier does not differ significantly from that published by Guillonneau and vallancien (2). The main difference is that these authors use interrupted sutures for urethrovesical anastomosis instead of a single circumferential running suture. First, they perform two sutures posteriorly at the 5 and 7 o'clock positions, inside-out on the urethra and outside-in on the bladder. These sutures are tied intraluminally. Four other sutures are then placed at the 4, 8, 2, and 10 o'clock positions, which are tied extraluminally. All these sutures are done forehand with the right needle holder: for right-sided sutures outside-in on the bladder and inside-out on the urethra, for left-sided sutures outside-in on the urethra and inside-out on the bladder. Finally, two anterior sutures are placed while the Foley catheter is inserted under visual control.

Both Guillonneau's and our technique, as well as later published procedures (3,4), are based on the primary access to the seminal vesicles, described originally by Kavoussi et al. (5).

In 1999, Rassweiler et al. (6) proposed a different laparoscopic technique derived from the classic retropubic radical prostatectomy. The intervention begins with immediate transperitoneal approach to Retzius's space. The dorsal vein complex and the urethra are divided, the endopelvic fascia incised, and the distal pedicles of the prostate transected. Then, the apex is pulled upward with the help of the sectioned Foley catheter, which facilitates the dissection between rectum and prostate. The bladder neck is incised. The vasa deferentia and seminal vesicles are reached transvesically. The vesicourethral anastomosis is performed with interrupted sutures.

Extraperitoneal endoscopic radical prostatectomy has been described and deserves mention (7). We have experience with this technique but find it moderately more difficult. We again use an open insertion technique for the initial umbilical trocar and locate the preperitoneal plane. A Foley catheter with a surgical glove is used as a balloon dissector to help create the prevesical space. We initially incise the endopelvic fascia and after dissecting the apex, secure the dorsal vein. Again, a second, more proximal, suture is used to retract the prostate anteriorly and aid in identifying the bladder neck. After dissecting and dividing the anterior bladder neck, the posterior bladder neck is divided sharply in the usual manner. Finding the seminal vesicles is slightly more difficult without them being dissected previously. Once found, they are easily dissected in a similar fashion to our transperitoneal approach. Denonvilliers' fascia is divided on its anterior surface and the rectoprostatic plane developed. The seminal vesicles are again used to expose the pedicles, which are divided prior to returning to the anterior side of the prostate to complete division of the dorsal vein and urethra. Once the specimen is placed in an endosac, depending on its size, it can interfere with the descent of the bladder, making the anastomosis more difficult. A 30° lens can be used to overcome this shortcoming.

PUBLISHED SERIES

The first radical prostatectomy performed via laparoscopy was reported by Schuessler et al. in 1992 (8). Initially, there was little enthusiasm for this new technique due to excessive operating times, no obvious benefits over traditional open surgery, and its perceived extreme difficulty. Even performed by an experienced team, the average operating time was 9.5 h, and this did not tend to decrease in the later patients. Several technical aspects remained unresolved, especially vesicourethral reconstruction, which required the greatest time and took twice as long as the removal of the prostate itself.

However, during the last 3 years laparoscopy has made a major comeback in the surgical treatment of localized prostate cancer. Several teams have succeeded in elaborating wholly standardized surgical procedures, which has led to a significant shortening of operating time. This has allowed introduction of laparoscopic radical prostatectomy in routine clinical use.

But for the laparoscopic approach to be adopted by the urologic community, it must offer at least comparable result with regard to oncologic control and morbidity. Large retrospective series of radical retropubic prostatectomy report varying continence rates from as low as 31% to as high as 92% (9,10). Variance can be explained by a number of factors including definitions of continence, methods of determination (physician interrogation vs. blinded patient reports), and physician experience. Furthermore, patient age and neurovascular bundle preservation have been demonstrated to correlate with return of urinary continence following radical retropubic prostatectomy (11). Potency also varies significantly with reported rates of 10% to as high as 86% among men undergoing nerve sparing procedures. Potency preservation has also been correlated well with patient age at surgery. Perioperative bleeding is highly variable as well, with some high-volume centers reporting averages of 1500 cc, whereas others have reported average rates under 500 cc with the use of a deep dorsal vein ligator (12).

A number of groups have now published their experiences with laparoscopic radical prostatectomy, and indeed it is replacing retropubic prostatectomy (Table 4.1). Guillonneau et al. (13) have published their experience with 350 patients. During their last 200 cases, operative time was ~195 min, average blood loss was 354 cc, and the transfusion rate was 2.8%. By the pathologic stage, the positive surgical margin rate was 3.6% for pT2a specimens, 14% for pT2b specimens, 33% for pT3a specimens, and 43.5% for pT34b specimens. Of the patients, 85.5% were pad free and 59% reported spontaneous return of erectile function following bilateral nerve sparing procedure.

Rassweiller et al. reported on 180 cases. Ninety-five percent of the patients did not require analgesics by postoperative day 2. Ninety-seven percent were continent at 1 year and positive margins were found in 16% of the specimens. Turk et al. (4) have reported on 145 procedures. Mean blood loss was 185 cc and 93% of the patients were continent at 6 months.

In our experience our transfusion rate is 2%. With at least 1 year of follow-up, 56% of the men reported erections (with or without sexual intercourse) without the use of Sildenafil. Diurnal and nocturnal urinary continence (no pads) was achieved in 86.2% and 100%, respectively, at 1 year. Average catheter time in our last 150 cases was <4 days.

ONCOLOGIC RESULTS

Our cancer control results were similar to those of conventional procedures; positive surgical margins were found in 24.6% of the patients. In a review of the literature, Wieder and Soloway (15) reported that the overall rate of a positive surgical margin with radical prostatectomy is 28% and that the apex was the most common location of tumor at the inked surface of the specimen. In a more recent study including 2518 patients, Blute et al. (16) reported an overall positive surgical margin rate of 39%, but the patients undergoing radical prostatectomy comprised also 10% of clinical stage T3 tumors. Therefore, the comparison of overall positive margin rates of different series may be strongly biased because of the dissimilarity of prostatectomy patient populations. The evaluation of the oncologic accuracy of the surgical excision is probably more balanced if we take into account only the pT2 specimens. In this respect, our 16.8% positive margin rate in organ-confined disease is satisfactory, considering the 26% positive margins found in a large series of open retropubic prostatectomies including 2712 pT2N0 patients (17).

ONCOLOGIC CONCERNS

The subject of oncologic risk specific to laparoscopic surgery in general is still controversial. Antagonists of this approach challenged that port site tumor

Table 4.1 Experiences with Laparoscopic Radical Prostatectomy

Series	Number of patients	Operating time	EBL (mL)	Transfusion rate (%)	Positive margins (%)	Continence at 12 months (%)	Erection with 2 NVB (%)	Conversions
Guillonneau et al. (13)	350	217	354	5.7	15.1 (pT2: 10.7)	85.5	59 at 6 months	7
Hozuck et al. (14)	217	285	783	2	24.6 (pT2:16.8)	86.2	56 at 1 year	0
Turk et al. (4)	145	255	185	2	24.5	93	NA	0
Rasweiller et al. (6)	180	271	NA	31	16	97	NA	5
Gill and Zippe (3)	40	336	340	2.5	23	NA	NA	1

Note: EBL, estimated blood loss; NVB, neuro-vascular bundles; NA, not available.

recurrence was intrinsic to laparoscopy (18,19). However, parietal metastases after laparoscopy were only anecdotal and mainly observed in gynecological and gastrointestinal cancers. More recently, several well-controlled clinical trials have shown that laparoscopic colectomy offers comparable oncologic results to open surgery (20).

With regard to prostate cancer, additional concern is raised over the transformation of a traditionally retropubic approach to one that is transperitoneal. However, based on currently available knowledge, prostate cancer does not belong to those neoplasms that have a high propensity for tumor seeding. Transrectal biopsy is the most common means of making a diagnosis of prostate cancer, yet documented biopsy tract tumor implantation is quite rare. While reports of local recurrence along the biopsy tract or along the needle track of a transperineal radioactive seed implantation do exist (21,22), these are largely in individual case reports. Haddad (23), in reviewing the literature on perineal biopsy, using larger tru-cut needles, found an incidence of only 0.4%. Many investigators have looked at the role of tumor cells liberated at the time of surgery to explain the phenomenon of local recurrence and Prostate-specific antigen (PSA) failure. Tumor cells have been detected in expressed seminal secretion from patients with pathologic T3 disease (24). Using more sensitive assays such as RT-PCR to detect PSA producing cells, investigators have shown 20 out of 22 patients with pathologic T2 disease to have evidence of "tumor spillage" in the operative field and 10 out of 22 patients had evidence of PSA producing cells in the peripheral blood during surgery (25). Similarly, older studies of men undergoing channel TURP have demonstrated transient circulating cancer cells, though well-matched studies of men undergoing TURP prior to radical prostatectomy have not demonstrated an increase in local or distant failure rates when compared to men diagnosed by traditional biopsy (26). It seems, therefore, that surgery on the prostate does indeed result in transient access of prostate cells to the circulation and that prostate cells likely are shed into the operative field during prostatectomy. The lack of correlation with local or distant failure, however, serves to underscore the contemporary understanding of the tumor cell. It is that simply releasing a tumor cell is not akin to metastasis and that the tumor cell needs to acquire the genetic potential for metastasis. Though long-term results are not available, it is unlikely that laparoscopy compromises the oncologic results of radical prostatectomy.

REFERENCES

1. Hoznek A, Salomon L, Rabii R, Ben Slama MR, Cicco A, Antiphon P, Abbou CC. Vesicourethral anastomosis during laparoscopic radical prostatectomy: the running suture method. J Endourol 2000; 14(9):749–753.
2. Guillonneau B, Vallancien G. Laparoscopic radical prostatectomy: the Montsouris technique. J Urol 2000; 163(6):1643–1649.

3. Gill IS, Zippe CD. Laparoscopic radical prostatectomy: technique. Urol Clin North Am 2001; 28(2):423–436.
4. Turk I, Deger IS, Winkelmann B, Roigas J, Schonberger B, Loening SA. Laparoscopic radical prostatectomy: experience with 145 procedures. Die laparoskopische radikale Prostatektomie. Erfahrungen mit 145 Eingriffen. Urol A 2001; 40(3):199–206.
5. Kavoussi LR, Schuessler WW, Vancaillie TG, Clayman RV. Laparoscopic approach to the seminal vesicles. J Urol 1993; 150(2 Pt 1):417–419.
6. Rassweiler J, Sentker L, Seemann O, Hatzinger M, Rumpelt H. Laparoscopic radical prostatectomy—the Heilbronn tehcnique: an analysis of the first 180 cases. J Urol 2001. In press.
7. Raboy A, Albert P, Ferzli G. Early experience with extraperitoneal endoscopic radical retropubic prostatectomy. Surg Endosc 1998; 12(10):1264–1267.
8. Schuessler WW, Schulam PG, Clayman RV, Kavoussi LR. Laparoscopic radical prostatectomy: initial short-term experience. Urology 1997; 50(6):854–857.
9. Bates TS, Wright MP, Gillatt DA. Prevalence and impact of incontinence and impotence following total prostatectomy assessed anonymously by the ICS-male questionnaire. Eur Urol 1998; 33(2):165–169.
10. Catalona WJ, Carvalhal GF, Mager DE, Smith DS. Potency, continence and complication rates in 1,870 consecutive radical retropubic prostatectomies. J Urol 1999; 162(2):433–438.
11. Wei JT, Dunn RL, Marcovich R, Montie JE, Sanda MG. Prospective assessment of patient reported urinary continence after radical prostatectomy. J Urol 2000; 164(3 Pt 1):744–748.
12. Avant OL, Jones JA, Beck H, Hunt C, Straub M. New method to improve treatment outcomes for radical prostatectomy. Urology 2000; 56(4):658–662.
13. Guillonneau B, Cathelineau X, Doublet JD, Vallancien G. Laparoscopic radical prostatectomy: the lessons learned. J Endourol 2001; 15(4):441–445.
14. Hoznek A, Salomon L, Olsson LE, Antiphon P, Saint F, Cicco A, Chopin D, Abbou CC. Laparoscopic radical prostatectomy: the Créteil experience. Eur Urol. In press.
15. Wieder JA, Soloway MS. Incidence, etiology, location, prevention and treatment of positive surgical margins after radical prostatectomy for prostate cancer. J Urol 1998; 160(2):299–315.
16. Blute ML, Bergstralh EJ, Iocca A, Scherer B, Zincke H. Use of Gleason score, prostate specific antigen, seminal vesicle and margin status to predict biochemical failure after radical prostatectomy. J Urol 2001; 165(1):119–125.
17. Blute ML, Bostwick DG, Bergstralh EJ, Slezak JM, Martin SK, Amling CL et al. Anatomic site-specific positive margins in organ-confined prostate cancer and its impact on outcome after radical prostatectomy. Urology 1997; 50(5):733–739.
18. Fusco MA, Paluzzi MW. Abdominal wall recurrence after laparoscopic-assisted colectomy for adenocarcinoma of the colon. Report of a case. Dis Colon Rectum 1993; 36(9):858–861.
19. Alexander RJ, Jaques BC, Mitchell KG. Laparoscopically assisted colectomy and wound recurrence. Lancet 1993; 341(8839):249–250.
20. Milsom JW, Bohm B, Hammerhofer KA, Fazio V, Steiger E, Elson P. A prospective, randomized trial comparing laparoscopic versus conventional techniques in colorectal cancer surgery: a preliminary report. J Am Coll Surg 1998; 187(1):46–54.

21. Moul JW, Bauer JJ, Srivastava S, Colon E, Ho CK, Sesterhenn IA et al. Perineal seeding of prostate cancer as the only evidence of clinical recurrence 14 years after needle biopsy and radical prostatectomy: molecular correlation. Urology 1998; 51(1):158–160.
22. Teh BS, Chou CC, Schwartz MR, Mai WY, Carpenter LS, Butler EB. Perineal prostatic cancer seeding following radioactive seed brachytherapy. J Urol 2001; 166(1):212.
23. Haddad FS. Re: risk factors for perineal seeding of prostate cancer after needle biopsy. J Urol 1990; 143(3):587–588.
24. Abi Aad AS, Noel H, Lorge F, Wese FX, Opsomer RJ, Van Cangh PJ. Do seminal or prostatic secretions play a role in local recurrence after radical prostatectomy for localized prostate cancer? Eur Urol 1993; 24(4):471–473.
25. Oefelein MG, Kaul K, Herz B, Blum MD, Holland JM, Keeler TC et al. Molecular detection of prostate epithelial cells from the surgical field and peripheral circulation during radical prostatectomy. J Urol 1996; 155(1):238–242.
26. Mansfield JT, Stephenson RA. Does transurethral resection of the prostate compromise the radical treatment of prostate cancer? Semin Urol Oncol 1996; 14(3):174–177.

5

Laparoscopic Nephrectomy for Renal Cell Carcinoma

Thomas H. S. Hsu

*Department of Urology, Stanford University School of Medicine,
Stanford, California, USA*

Louis R. Kavoussi

*James Buchanan Brady Urological Institute,
Johns Hopkins Medical Institute, Baltimore, Maryland, USA*

INTRODUCTION

Renal cell carcinoma (RCC) accounts for ~3% of all adult malignancies, and 23,000 to 28,000 new cases are diagnosed in the USA each year (1,2). Surgical resection has been the most effective management to cure localized RCC, and radical nephrectomy has long been considered as the gold-standard (1). Radical nephrectomy requires en bloc removal of the affected kidney with the enveloping Gerota's fascia.

The first laparoscopic nephrectomy performed by Clayman and Co-workers in 1990 led the way to the establishment of this technique as a viable alternative to open surgery in the management of benign renal diseases (3,4). Several investigators have confirmed that laparoscopic nephrectomy provides decreased postoperative morbidity, optimal cosmetic results, and faster convalescence when compared with traditional approaches (5,6).

Laparoscopic nephrectomy for localized RCC was initially controversial due to concerns of local recurrence, adequate cancer control, and risk of port-site seeding (7–13). However, reports on laparoscopic radical nephrectomy for RCC from various centers not only confirmed the benefits of laparoscopy but also demonstrated the safety and oncologic efficacy of the laparoscopic procedure for RCC on a short-term basis (14–17). These early reports provided much optimism and interest in the development of laparoscopic nephrectomy for RCC, and to date, hundreds of laparoscopic radical nephrectomies for RCC have been performed at centers worldwide (18,19).

This chapter is a current review of the literature and attempts to present an overview of the most commonly used surgical techniques for laparoscopic radical nephrectomy, preoperative and postoperative preparation, as well as recent results and complication data. Finally, the current, yet very limited, data on laparoscopic partial nephrectomy for RCC will be discussed.

INDICATIONS AND CONTRAINDICATIONS

Indications for laparoscopic radical nephrectomy for RCC have changed significantly over the last few years, and the general accepted indications in most centers at this time are $T_1-T_2N_0M_0$ tumors <10 cm in size (20). However, size and stage are not absolute indications and application. This technique should be individualized for each patient and surgeon's experience. Indeed, there have been successful reports of cases with level 1 renal vein thrombus, T_4 (locally invasive) tumors, and distant metastases as part of cytoreductive immunotherapy protocol (S. J. Savage and I. S. Gill, unpublished data) (21,22). Wider applications will continue to expand with increasing experience in this procedure.

General contraindications to laparoscopic radical nephrectomy are similar to those previously described for most abdominal laparoscopic procedures (23). These include inability to tolerate general anesthesia, severe cardiopulmonary disease unfit for surgery, uncorrected coagulopathy, and hypovolemic shock.

PREOPERATIVE PATIENT EVALUATION AND PREPARATION

Routine laboratory studies are conducted preoperatively as indicated. Preoperative metastatic evaluation for renal malignancy usually includes chest X-ray and computerized tomography (CT) of abdomen and pelvis. Bone scan is obtained if the patient experiences bone pain or has elevated serum alkaline phosphatase or serum calcium. MRI may be obtained if there is a suspicion of inferior vena cava involvement. In addition, CT of brain is recommended if the patient experiences seizures or other neurologic symptoms.

A detailed informed consent addressing the risks of laparoscopy (including hypercarbia and open conversion), the risks of nephrectomy (including hemorrhage and injury to adjacent organs or tissues), and the risks and modalities of blood replacement should be obtained from the patient before the surgery. Preoperative bowel preparation is done at the discretion of the surgeon. The patient is asked to have nothing by mouth after midnight prior to surgery. Type and screen are obtained, with cross-matching done on an individual basis. Intravenous broad-spectrum antibiotics such as cefazolin are administered on call to the operating room.

TECHNIQUES

Transperitoneal Approach

Several popular transperitoneal laparoscopic nephrectomy techniques have been previously described (20,23,24). Urethral Foley catheter and orogastric tube are routinely employed. The patient is placed in the flank or modified flank position. Ample padding of soft tissues and bony sites, including the head, neck, hip, knees, and ankles, and adequate support of the neck, arms, and legs must be ensured to prevent neuromuscular injury. Patients also need to be adequately secured to the table to prevent movement when tilting the bed.

At our institution, a three-port approach is typically used (Fig. 5.1). Following CO_2 insufflation of the peritoneal cavity with a Veress needle to 20 mmHg, a 12 mm Visiport trocar (US Surgical, Norwalk, CT) is placed at the level of the umbilicus, lateral to the ipsilateral rectus muscle. A 12 mm port (camera port)

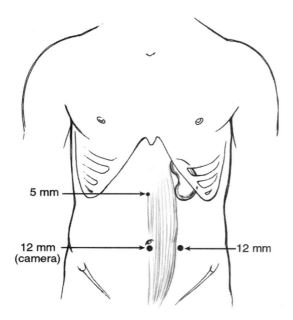

Figure 5.1   Trocar placement of transperitoneal laparoscopic radical nephrectomy.

is placed at the umbilicus, and a 5 mm port is placed at the midpoint between the umbilicus and the xiphoid process.

Alternatively, a four- to five-port approach initially described by Dunn et al. (20) can be used. Through a 12 mm incision two fingerbreadths above and two fingerbreadths medial to the anterior superior iliac spine, initial access to the peritoneal cavity may be obtained using a Veress needle or the Hasson cannula technique. Following insufflation of the peritoneal cavity, additional ports are placed as follows: a 12 mm port two to three fingerbreadths supraumbilically and in the midclavicular/pararectus line (for a 10 mm laparoscope), a 12 mm port two fingerbreadths subcostally in the anterior axillary line, and a 5 mm port two fingerbreadths subcostally in the midaxillary line. Additionally, a 5 mm port in the midaxillary line just above the iliac crest may be placed to facilitate kidney specimen entrapment, and a 5 mm port two fingerbreadths below the xiphoid process in the midline may be placed to allow liver retraction during right renal hilar dissection.

Following successful trocar placement, peritoneal incision of the line of Toldt is first performed to allow medial mobilization of the colon. The caudal extension of the peritoneal incision is the common iliac artery, and the cranial extension is approximately above the hepatic or splenic flexure and includes the hepatic triangular ligament during a right nephrectomy and lienorenal and phrenicocolic ligaments during a left nephrectomy. The plane between the anterior Gerota's fascia and colonic mesentery can be identified once colorenal attachments are transected. In a right-sided procedure, a Kocher maneuver is then performed to reflect the duodenum and expose the anterior aspect of the inferior vena cava. For a left-sided procedure, the spleen is mobilized medially away from the left kidney. Following mobilization, the anterior surface of the kidney within the intact Gerota's fascia and the renal hilum should be fully exposed.

Upon inspection of the renal hilar region, the gonadal vein can be identified and traced proximally to identify the renal vein on the left, where it is clip ligated and divided. The left adrenal vein draining into the renal vein may also be ident-ified at this time, which is similarly clip ligated and transected. The ureter can be identified along the medial aspect of the renal specimen, and lateral ureteral retraction places the renal hilum on gentle stretch, facilitating hilar dissection. The renal vein is usually identified before the artery, which is commonly pos-terior and superior to the vein. The renal artery is first circumferentially dissected, clip ligated, and transected. Following arterial transection, the renal vein should appear flat. If the renal vein remains engorged, accessory renal arteries need to be sought and ligated prior to renal vein ligation. The vein is then circumferentially mobilized and transected with Endo-GIA vascular stapler.

A technique of rapid ligation of renal hilum for transperitoneal laparoscopic nephrectomy was recently described by Chan et al. (24). This technique does not require complete skeletonization of the renal vein or artery. Based on is technique, once the inferior edge of the renal vein is identified, the space between the vein and the posterior tissue encasing the renal artery is opened with a blunt laparoscopic grasper. As the space gives way, the grasper is advanced further behind the renal vein. Once an adequate space (of at least 2–3 cm in distance) is developed behind the vein, an Endo-GIA vascular stapler can be inserted to ligate the renal artery and surrounding lymphatics within the posterior tissue. Once the renal vein has collapsed, it is similarly ligated and divided with the Endo-GIA stapler. This technique, successfully performed in over 100 patients, can help reduce the oper-ating time by ~10–15 min and may help reduce inadvertent vascular injuries.

Following hilar control, the kidney within the intact Gerota's fascia is then mobilized circumferentially. It is important to ensure that a sufficiently cephalad incision in the peritoneal reflection is made to allow the liver (in right nephrect-omy) or spleen (in left nephrectomy) to be displaced medially, thereby facilitating dissection and mobilization of the upper pole of the specimen. Gentle, atraumatic retraction of the liver/spleen may be helpful. The adrenal gland is usually spared, except in cases with large upper pole renal tumors. If adenalectomy is to be performed, the adrenal vessels need to be meticulously clip ligated and divided.

After the kidney within the intact Gerota's fascia has been completely mobilized from the surrounding tissues, the ureter is identified, clip ligated, and transected. The specimen is then entrapped in an Endocatch bag (US Surgical, Norwalk, CT) or a Lapsac (Cook Urological, Spencer, IN). Entrapment of the tumor specimen prior to its removal prevents possible wound contamination. The entrapped specimen can then be extracted intact via an extension of an existing port incision (most commonly the periumbilical port) or via a lower midline or Pfannenstiel incision. Alternatively, the specimen can be morcellated mechanically by forceps or electrically by a tissue morcellator without enlarging the existing port incisions, followed by specimen removal. Laboratory studies have demonstrated that as long as the entrapment sack is not punctured, it remains impermeable, thereby preventing tumor spillage, during morcellation (25). Morcellation can affect pathologic staging; however, this currently does not impact on the postoperative management of RCC.

At the conclusion of the surgical procedure, the pneumoperitoneum is lowered, and a complete and careful inspection of the retroperitoneum, adjacent soft tissues, and trocar sites is performed to ensure hemostasis. Fascial defects of >5 mm trocars are closed, and incisional sites are reapproximated with absorbable sutures. No surgical drain is necessary.

Hand-Assisted Transperitoneal Approach

The method commonly used in hand-assisted transperitoneal nephrectomy has been that described at several centers (26–28).

The patient is placed in a full or modified flank position, with adequate padding and support to various pressure points. The hand-assisted device (Intromit, Applied Medical, Santa Margarita, CA; PneumoSleeve, Pilling Weck, Inc., Research Triangle Park, NC; Handport, Smith and Nephew, Andover, MA) is typically placed at a supraumbilical midline incision (Fig. 5.2), the size of

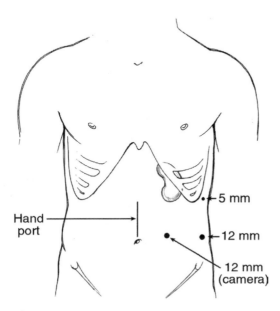

Figure 5.2 Trocar placement of hand-assisted transperitoneal laparoscopic radical nephrectomy.

which is equal to the surgeon's glove size in centimeters. After establishing the pneumoperitoneum, two ports are usually placed. A 12 mm camera port is placed in the midclavicular line lateral to the ipsilateral rectus muscle and slightly above the umbilicus. A 12 mm instrument port is placed in the midaxillary line at the level of the umbilicus. A second (5 or 12 mm) instrument port may be placed along the midaxillary line subcostally for retraction.

The surgeon inserts the nondominant hand through the hand-assisted device and performs fine surgical maneuvers with the dominant hand through the 12 mm instrument port. The back of the nondominant hand is frequently used as a retractor for liver/spleen during dissection and mobilization of the upper pole of the kidney. The general steps and laparoscopic instruments for hand-assisted laparoscopic nephrectomy are similar to those described for the standard transperitoneal approach above. At the end of the procedure, the specimen can be retrieved intact via the midline incision for the hand-assisted device.

Retroperitoneal Approach

Retroperitoneal laparoscopic nephrectomy was first described at Washington University in 1993 (29). This has been modified by several investigators since (30,31). The patient is securely placed in the full flank position. Elevation of the kidney rest and flexion of the operating table are performed to maximize the space between the lowermost rib and the iliac crest, as during open nephrectomy via the flank approach. All bony prominences and pressure points are carefully padded with egg-crate foam. Extremities are carefully placed in a neutral position to minimize the risk of neuromuscular injury.

The Hasson open technique is the typical access method to the retroperitoneal space. A 1.5 to 2 cm incision is made just below the tip of the 12th rib. Entry into the retroperitoneum is achieved by gently piercing the anterior throacolumbar fascia with the fingertip or a hemostat. Remaining anterior to the psoas fascia and posterior to the Gerota's fascia, gentle finger dissection of the retroperitoneum creates an initial retroperitoneal working space. An adequate working space in the retroperitoneum is then created by a balloon dilator device (Origin Medsystems, Menlo Park, CA) inflated with ~800 mL of air. The distended balloon displaces the kidney and Gerota's fascia anteromedially, which allows access to the posterior aspect of the renal hilum.

A 10 or 12 mm laparoscopic trocar is placed as the camera port after deflation and removal of the balloon device. Pneumoretroperitoneum of 15 mmHg is created, and the placement of two–three secondary ports (instrument ports) is done (Fig. 5.3), with laparoscopic or digital monitoring. A posterior port is placed at the angle between the 12th rib and the lateral border of the erector spinae muscles. An anterior port is placed 2–3 cm cephalad to the iliac crest, between the mid- and the anterior axillary lines. Either of the two secondary ports can be 5 or 10 mm. Occasionally, a fourth port (5 mm), located at the tip of the 11th rib in the anterior axillary line, may be needed for retraction purposes.

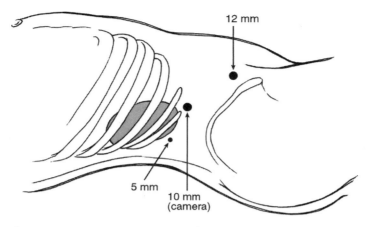

Figure 5.3   Trocar placement of retroperitoneal laparoscopic radical nephrectomy.

The search for renal arterial pulsations in the hilar region and dissection of the overlying fat lead to identification of the renal artery. The artery is mobilized, clip ligated, and transected. The more anteriorly located renal vein is then identified, mobilized, stapled, and divided with an Endo-GIA stapler. Its adrenal or gonadal branches may also need to be clip ligated and divided at this time.

The kidney within the intact Gerota's fascia is then circumferentially mobilized. Meticulous hemostasis is maintained at all times. The ureter is then clipped and divided. The freed specimen is placed within the Endocatch bag, which is typically removed intact through an extension of one of the posterior port sites. Further enlargement of the port site with a scalpel is often needed for larger specimens.

At the end of the procedure the pneumoretroperitoneum is lowered to confirm hemostasis in the retroperitoneum and the port sites. After hemostasis is ensured, incisional sites are closed with surgical sutures. No surgical drain is necessary.

POSTOPERATIVE PATIENT MANAGEMENT

Orogastric tube is removed at the end of the surgery. In general, urethral Foley catheter removal and resumption of oral intake and ambulation occur within the first 24 h. Parenteral and oral antibiotics are usually continued for the first few days postoperatively. Pain control can be achieved via routine parenteral or oral analgesics. Postoperative abdominal pain that is out of proportion to the skin incision size may suggest intra-abdominal organ injury. If bowel injury or any other intra-abdominal complication is suspected, appropriate radiologic and serologic studies need to be done.

RESULTS

Transperitoneal Approach

Transperitoneal laparoscopic nephrectomy for RCC has been performed success-fully at several centers worldwide. In a recent review by Ono et al. (32), 60 patients underwent laparoscopic radical nephrectomy for RCC ≤ 5 cm between 1992 and 1998. Mean operating time was 5.2 h, with mean blood loss of 255 mL, mean specimen weight of 279 g, mean analgesic use of 43 mg of penta-zocine, and mean time to full convalescence of 23 days. With a median follow-up of 24 months, two (3%) patients had distant metastasis without local recurrence or port-site seeding. Compared to the contemporary open group ($N = 40$), the laparoscopic group ($n = 60$) was found to have a significantly longer operating time, lower blood loss, and faster convalescence. Five-year disease-free survival between open and laparoscopic groups was not significantly different (97.5% and 95.5%, respectively; $p = $ NS).

Based on 72 laparoscopic radical nephrectomy patients for solid renal masses, Barrett et al. (33) reported mean operating time of 175 min, average specimen weight of 402.5 g, and mean hospital stay of 4.4 days. Fifty-seven of the 72 patients were found to have RCC on pathologic analysis. With a longer mean follow-up of 33.4 months on the same 57 patients, the Canadian group recently reported 5% (3/57) metastasis rate: one patient with local renal fossa recurrence and pulmonary metastasis, one with pulmonary and bone metastases, and one with solitary port-site recurrence on the abdominal wall (34). There was no apparent breakdown in the operating technique in the case of wound seeding, which represents the only reported case of local trocar-site recurrence after laparoscopic nephrectomy for RCC in the literature.

In a recent review by Clayman's group (35), 61 patients underwent trans-peritoneal laparoscopic nephrectomy for suspected RCC from 1990 to 1998, with 47 patients diagnosed with RCC on pathology. Mean operating time was 5.5 h. Mean estimated blood loss was 172 mL. Average analgesic requirement was 27 mg morphine sulfate equivalent, and mean hospital stay was 3.6 days. Average times to normal activity and 100% recovery were 3.8 and 8.4 weeks, respectively. Compared to the open nephrectomy data from the same institution, the laparoscopic group had a statistically significant longer operating time but lower blood loss, lower postoperative analgesic need, shorter hospital stay, and faster convalescence. With a mean follow-up of 28 months, 13% patients in the laparoscopic group (vs. 10% in the open group) developed tumor recurrence without trocar or intraoperitoneal seeding.

Chan et al. (36) recently reported their experience from the standpoint of cancer control. Sixty-seven patients underwent laparoscopic radical nephrectomy from 1991 to 1999 for clinically localized, pathologically confirmed $T_1-T_2N_0M_0$ RCC. With a mean follow-up of 35.6 months, there was no laparoscopic port-site or renal fossa tumor recurrence. No significant difference was found in the Kaplan Meier disease-free survival and actuarial survival analysis between the laparoscopic radical nephrectomy group and its contemporary open cohort ($N = 54$).

Complications of Standard Transperitoneal Approach

In an earlier multi-institutional review of patients undergoing laparoscopic radical nephrectomy for renal malignancies, complications occurred in 34% patients (37). With experience, complication rates decreased. In a more recent multi-institutional review, the overall complication was found to be 23% (7% major and 16% minor), with open conversion rate of 4% (18).

In the series of 72 patients with transperitoneal laparoscopic radical nephrectomy reported by Barrett et al. (33), there were two (2.7%) intraoperative complications (including polar artery bleeding in one patient and minor splenic injury in one) and seven (9.7%) postoperative complications (including blood transfusion in two, ileus/bowel obstruction in three, wound infection in one, and unstable angina in one). In the updated series of 60 patients undergoing laparoscopic radical nephrectomy for RCC in Ono et al. (32), there was one open conversion due to renal artery bleeding requiring nephrectomy. In addition, there were five (8.3%) intraoperative complications (including renal artery injury in one patient, splenic injury in one, adrenal injury in one, periureteral artery injury in one, and duodenal injury in one) and three (5%) postoperative complications (including paralytic ileus in two patients and pulmonary embolism in one). Compared to the open cohort of 40 patients, there was no significant difference in the complication rate. This finding was also supported by a recent update from Clayman's group of 61 laparoscopic patients, demonstrating that the intraoperative and postoperative complication rates did not significantly differ between the laparoscopic and open groups (20,38).

Hand-Assisted Transperitoneal Approach

A report by Wolf et al. (27) on three hand-assisted radical nephrectomies for RCC showed mean operating time of 231 min, mean blood loss of 192 mL, and mean specimen weight of 271 g. Shichman et al. (39) reported 19 hand-assisted radical nephrectomies for preoperatively diagnosed renal masses over a 6 month period. Mean operating time was 219 min, with mean estimated blood loss of 203.6 mL, mean hospital stay of 3.5 days, and mean postoperative narcotic requirement of 34.5 mg morphine sulfate equivalent. All specimens were extracted intact without morcellation or violation of Gerota's fascia.

Fadden and Nakada (28) recently reported short-term data on 17 hand-assisted radical nephrectomies. Mean operating time was 222 min, and mean estimated blood loss was 171 mL. Mean hospitalization was 3.9 days, and mean time to normal activity was 16 days. Further long-term data on cancer control are still pending.

Complications of Hand-Assisted Transperitoneal Approach

Shichman et al. (39) reported a 6.6% complication rate in their group of 19 patients undergoing hand-assisted laparoscopic radical nephrectomy. No open conversion was reported in the series from Shichman et al. (39), Wolf et al. (27), or Fadden and Nakada (28).

Retroperitoneal Approach

Abbou et al. (40) reported data on 29 patients undergoing retroperitoneal laparoscopic nephrectomy for renal tumors from 1995 to 1998. Compared to the contemporary open group, the laparoscopic group had a mean operating time of 145 min (vs. 121 min in the open group; $p = 0.047$), mean blood loss of 100 mL (vs. 284 mL; $p < 0.005$), mean parenteral narcotic requirement of 1.8 mg morphine sulfate (vs. 3.2 mg; $p < 0.05$), mean hospital stay of 4.8 days (vs. 9.7 days; $p < 0.001$), and mean tumor size of 4 cm (vs. 5.7 cm; $p < 0.005$). In the laparoscopic group, pathologic staging revealed pT_1 RCC in 7 patients, pT_2 in 10, and pT_3 in 8, with negative surgical margins in all cases. With a mean follow-up of 15 months, local recurrence with hepatitic metastasis occurred in one (3.4%) laparoscopic group patient.

Gill (18) reported a retroperitoneal laparoscopic radical nephrectomy series comprising more than 85 patients. Of the first 53 cases, the average surgical time was 2.9 h, with mean blood loss of 128 mL, mean specimen weight of 484 g, mean tumor size of 4.6 cm, and mean hospital stay of 1.6 days. On histology, 42 of 53 cases were diagnosed with RCC, all of which were with negative surgical margins. Pathologic staging revealed pT_1 in 36, pT_2 in 4, pT_{3a} in 1, and pT_{3b} in 1. With a mean follow-up of 13 months, there was no recurrence in renal fossa/port sites or cancer-specific mortality; however, two patients with pT_1 RCC developed metastases between 8 and 12 months postoperatively. The safety, efficacy, and minimal patient morbidity provided by the retroperitoneal laparoscopic radical nephrectomy in the octogenarian/nonagenarian population and high-risk patient population have also been demonstrated by Hsu et al. (41, unpublished data).

Complications of Retroperitoneal Approach

Abbou et al. (40) reported a 6.8% complication rate in their 29 retroperitoneal laparoscopic radical nephrectomy cases. In this series, two complications occurred—including one case of colon injury requiring temporary colostomy and one case of massive bleeding due to renal artery staple dislodgment during specimen removal, which required open conversion and blood transfusion. Compared to a contemporary open radical nephrectomy cohort, the laparoscopic group was found to have a significantly lower complication rate (24% vs. 8%, respectively).

In his initial 53 cases, Gill (18) reported major complications in two (4%) patients and minor complications in eight (17%). The major complications were renal vein injury in one and clip dislodgment from a renal arterial branch in one, both of which were controlled by open conversion. The minor complications included superficial port-site infection, peri-incisional parethesia, and self-limiting retroperitoneal hematoma.

COMPARISON OF THE VARIOUS LAPAROSCOPIC TECHNIQUES

All previously discussed approaches, both transperitoneal and retroperitoneal, can provide efficacious and safe surgical removal of renal malignancies. Thus far in the literature, no death has been associated with laparoscopic radical nephrectomy. The optimal surgical approach depends on the individual clinical situations (such as previous abdominal or retroperitoneal surgeries) and, more importantly, the surgeon's previous training and personal experience.

The transperitoneal approach provides a large working space, easier identification of colon and other relevant anatomic landmarks, and easier specimen mobilization and entrapment within the larger peritoneal space. The hand-assisted approach further provides tactile sensation, depth perception, and a much lower learning curve (39). The hand-assisted approach is associated with a larger incision from the hand-assisted device placement.

The retroperitoneal approach provides rapid access to the renal hilum (18,42). However, it is associated with a significantly smaller working space, less evident anatomic landmarks, and more difficult organ entrapment.

LAPAROSCOPIC PARTIAL NEPHRECTOMY FOR RCC

Overview of Techniques

The surgical approach to the kidney is identical to that for laparoscopic radical nephrectomy and can be either transperitoneal or retroperitoneal. Use of laparoscopic ultrasound probe may facilitate identifying the exact location and depth of the renal tumor. Vascular control of the main renal vessels can be achieved via Roummell tourniquet or laparoscopic vascular bulldog clamps (43–48). Parenchymal incision may be performed with Harmonic Scalpel (Ethicon Endo-surgery, Inc., Cincinnati, OH) or monopolar/bipolar electrocautery (49,50). Injury to the collecting system can be identified with the use of indigo carmine and needs to be suture repaired. Topical fibrin glue, oxidized cellulose (Oxycel, Becton Dickinson and Company, Franklin Lakes, NJ), and/or argon beam laser may be applied to the resection surface for hemostasis (49–52). Through an existing trocar incision, a drain is usually placed near the resection site, as in open partial nephrectomy. A stent is rarely utilized.

Clinical Results

Current experiences have been limited to small (<3–4 cm), exophytic renal tumors (49,50,53,54). Winfield's group (49) reported three laparoscopic wedge resections for exophytic renal tumors ≤3 cm in size, with operating time of <3.5 h, no open conversion, and hospitalization of <3 days.

Janetschek et al. (50) reported seven laparoscopic wedge resections for exophytic renal tumors ≤2 cm in size. Operating time ranged from 2.5 to 5 h, and blood loss ranged from 190 to 800 mL. Postoperatively, serum creatinine was unchanged. Pneumothorax in one patient was the only complication, which resolved spontaneously. Five patients were pathologically diagnosed with RCC. With a mean follow-up of 18 months, there was no local recurrence or distant metastasis.

Abbou's group (54) reported 13 cases of retroperitoneal laparoscopic wedge resection. The three patients pathologically diagnosed with RCC had median operating time of 180 min, median warm ischemia time of 10 min, median blood loss of 200 mL, and median hospitalization of 5 days. Postoperative complication of urinary leak occurred in one patient.

A multicenter European experience of laparoscopic wedge resection of tumors with average size of 2.3 cm was recently reported by Rassweiler et al. (55). A total of 53 patients underwent laparoscopic partial nephrectomy from 1994 to 2000, with mean operating time of 191 min, mean blood loss of 725 mL, 8% open conversion rate, mean hospital stay of 5.4 days, and six (11.3%) postoperative complications (rebleeding in one patient and urinoma in five) requiring reintervention. Histology showed 37 (69%) cases of RCC, which had 100% survival at 3 years.

Bishoff and Kavoussi (56) described their laparoscopic nephron-sparing nephrectomy for clinically T_1 solid renal masses (mean size 2.3 cm) in a recent report. Twenty-four patients underwent the laparoscopic surgery successfully, with mean operating time of 155 min and blood loss of 265 mL. Mean hospital stay was 2.6 days. Twenty (83%) patients were found to have RCC histologically, and all these cases had negative surgical margins. Complications included pneumothorax (one patient) and need for urine drainage with stent or Jackson-Pratt drain (three patients). At a mean follow-up of 7.3 months, there was no tumor recurrence or port-site seeding.

The Cleveland Clinic experience of laparoscopic partial nephrectomy was recently reported by Gill's group (57). All 36 cases were completed successfully with a mean operating time of 2.9 h, warm ischemia time of 20.5 min, and blood loss of 237 mL. Mean hospital stay was 1.7 days. Complications included blood transfusion (one patient), inadvertent enterotomy requiring suture repair (one), atelectasis (one), and atrial fibrillation (one). There was no urine leak postoperatively. Final histology showed 20 (56%) cases of RCC, and all surgical margins were negative for cancer.

CONCLUSIONS

Laparoscopic radical nephrectomy has evolved into an established treatment modality for RCC. Compared to open surgery, it has been shown to be equally safe and, furthermore, can provide patients with decreased postoperative morbidity and more rapid convalescence. The choice of transperitoneal vs. retroperitoneal approach is primarily dependent on the surgeon's preference and patient's history, as there are good outcome data supporting both techniques. There is a steep learning curve associated with standard transperitoneal and retroperitoneal techniques, but operating time can decrease with increasing operator experience (20). Hand-assisted laparoscopy is more easily learned and may be more readily applied by the community urologist (28).

Laparoscopic radical nephrectomy as an oncologic procedure for RCC has been shown to be efficacious, as discussed previously. This view is further supported by a recent multi-institutional study, in which laparoscopic nephrectomy (both transperitoneal and retroperitoneal) for localized RCC in 157 patients was found to have 2.5% (4/157) distant metastasis but no port-site or renal fossa recurrence postoperatively at a mean follow-up of 19 months (58). Distant metastasis and renal fossa/retroperitoneal recurrence, although not common, can occur after laparoscopic radical nephrectomy, and the findings are consistent with the natural history of RCC (59). In fact, the short-term and intermediate-term laparoscopic radical nephrectomy data from various centers presented earlier compared favorably with those of the open radical nephrectomy reports: 13–14% local/retroperitoneal recurrence in the pre-CT era, 32–37% local recurrence in the post-CT era, and up to 50% metachronous metastasis after open radical nephrectomy with curative intent (60–63). Port-site recurrence after laparoscopic procedure is rare, with only two reported cases in the literature (34,64). Specimen retrieval at the end of laparoscopic nephrectomy needs to be performed meticulously and carefully to avoid local wound seeding.

In sum, all the available data from various laparoscopic centers have shown that laparoscopic radical nephrectomy is a viable treatment option for select patients with RCC. A large amount of long-term (5 year and 10 year) laparoscopic data for RCC is still pending.

Laparoscopic partial nephrectomy is technically more challenging from the hemostatic and reconstructive perspectives, and current clinical data are limited. Novel modalities for parenchymal resection and hemostasis are being developed (50,65). Further clinical experience will help to define its role in the management of RCC.

REFERENCES

1. Belldegrun A, deKernion JB. Renal tumors. In: Walsh PC, Retik AB, Vaughn ED, Wein AJ, eds. Campbell's Urology. Philadelphia: W.B. Saunders Company, 1998:2283–2326.
2. Eble JN. Neoplasms of the kidney. In: Bostwick DG, Eble JN, eds. Urologic Surgical Pathology. St. Louis: Mosby, 1997:83–148.
3. Clayman RV, Kavoussi LR, Soper NJ. Laparoscopic nephrectomy. N Engl J Med 1991; 324:1370–1371.

4. Clayman RV, Kavoussi LR, Soper NJ. Laparoscopic nephrectomy: initial case report. J Urol 1991; 146:278–282.
5. Coptcoat M, Joyce A, Rassweiler J, Popert R. Laparoscopic nephrectomy: the Kings clinical experience. J Urol 1992; 147:433A.
6. Kerbl K, Clayman RV, McDougall EM, Kavoussi LR. Laparoscopic nephrectomy: the Washington University experience. Br J Urol 1994; 73:231–236.
7. Ramos JM, Gupta S, Anthone GJ. Laparoscopy and colon cancer: is the port site at risk? A preliminary report. Arch Surg 1994; 129:897–900.
8. Childers JM, Aqua KA, Surwit EA. Abdominal-wall tumor implantation after laparoscopy for malignant conditions. Obstet Gynecol 1994; 84:765–769.
9. Cirrocco WC, Schwartzman A, Golub RW. Abdominal-wall recurrence after laparoscopic colectomy for colon cancer. Surgery 1994; 116:842–846.
10. Nduka CC, Monson JRT, Menzies-Gow N. Abdominal-wall metastases following laparoscopy. Br J Surg 1994; 81:648–652.
11. Johnstone PA, Rohde DC, Swartz SE. Port site recurrences after laparoscopic and thoracoscopic procedures in malignancy. J Clin Oncol 1996; 14:1950–1956.
12. Andersen JR, Steven K. Implantation metastasis after laparoscopic biopsy of bladder cancer. J Urol 1995; 153:1047–1048.
13. Bangma CH, Kirkels WJ, Chadha S. Cutaneous metastasis following laparoscopic pelvic lymphadenectomy for prostate carcinoma. J Urol 1995; 153:1635–1636.
14. Rassweiler J, Henkel TO, Potempa DM, Coptcoat MJ, Miller K, Preminger GM, Alken P. Transperitoneal laparoscopic nephrectomy: training, technique, and results. J Endourol 1993; 7:505–514.
15. Kavoussi LR, Kerbl K, Capelouto CC, McDougall EM, Clayman RV. Laparoscopic nephrectomy for renal neoplasms. Urology 1993; 42:603–609.
16. Ono Y, Sahashi M, Yamada S, Ohshima S. Laparoscopic nephrectomy without morcellation for renal cell carcinoma: report of initial 2 cases. J Urol 1993; 150:1222–1224.
17. Ono Y, Katoh N, Kinukawa T, Sahashi M, Ohshima S. Laparoscopic nephrectomy, radical nephrectomy and adrenalectomy: Nagoya experience. J Urol 1994; 152:1962–1966.
18. Gill IS. Laparoscopic radical nephrectomy for cancer. Urol Clin North Am 2000; 27:707–719.
19. Schulam PG, deKernion JB. Laparoscopic nephrectomy for renal cell carcinoma: the current situation. J Endourol 2001; 15:375–376.
20. Dunn MD, McDougall EM, Clayman RV. Laparoscopic radical nephrectomy. J Endourol 2000; 14:849–858.
21. Savage SJ, Gill IS. Laparoscopic radical nephrectomy for renal cell carcinoma with preoperatively staged level I renal vein tumor thrombus. J Urol 2000; 163:1243–1244.
22. Walher MM, Lyne JC, Libutti SK. Laparoscopic cytoreductive nephrectomy as preparation for administration of systemic interleukin 2 in the treatment of metastatic renal cell carcinoma: a pilot study. Urology 1999; 53:496–499.
23. Peters C, Kavoussi LR. Laparoscopy in children and adults. In: Walsh PC, Retik AB, Vaughn ED, Wein AJ, eds. Campbell's Urology. Philadelphia: W.B. Saunders Company, 1998:2875–2912.
24. Chan DY, Su L, Kavoussi LR. Rapid ligation of renal hilum during transperitoneal laparoscopic nephrectomy. Urology 2001; 57:360–362.

25. Urban DA, Kerbl K, McDougall EM, Stone AM, Fadden PT, Clayman RV. Organ entrapment and renal morcellation: permeability studies. J Urol 1993; 150:1792–1794.
26. Wolf JS, Moon TD, Nakada SY. Hand assisted laparoscopic nephrectomy: technical considerations. Tech Urol 1997; 3:123–128.
27. Wolf JS, Moon TD, Nakada SY. Hand assisted laparoscopic nephrectomy: comparison to standard laparoscopic nephrectomy. J Urol 1998; 160:22–27.
28. Fadden PT, Nakada SY. Hand-assisted laparoscopic renal surgery. Urol Clin North Am 2001; 28:167–176.
29. Kerbl K, Figenshau RS, Clayman RV, Chandhoke PS, Kavoussi LR, Stone AM. Retroperitoneal laparoscopic nephrectomy: laboratory and clinical experience. J Endourol 1993; 7:23–26.
30. Gill IS. Retroperitoneal laparoscopic nephrectomy. Urol Clin North Am 1998; 25:343–360.
31. Hsu TH, Sung GT, Gill IS. Retroperitoneoscopic approach to nephrectomy. J Endourol 1999; 13:713–720.
32. Ono Y, Kinukawa T, Hattori R, Yamada S, Nishiyama N, Mizutani K, Ohshima S. Laparoscopic radical nephrectomy for renal cell carcinoma: a five-year experience. Urology 1999; 53:280–286.
33. Barrett PH, Fentie DD, Taranger LA. Laparoscopic radical nephrectomy with morcellation for renal cell carcinoma: the Saskatoon experience. Urology 1998; 52:23–28.
34. Fentie DD, Barrett PH, Taranger LA. Metastatic renal cell cancer after laparoscopic radical nephrectomy: long-term follow-up. J Endourol 2000; 14:407–411.
35. Dunn MD, Portis AJ, Shalhav AL, Elbahnasy AM, McDougall EM, Clayman RV. Laparoscopic versus open radical nephrectomy for renal tumor: the Washington University experience. J Urol 1999; 161:166A.
36. Chan DY, Cadeddu JA, Jarrett TW, Marshall FF, Kavoussi LR. Laparoscopic radical nephrectomy: cancer control in renal cell carcinoma. J Urol 2001; 166:2095–2099.
37. Gill IS, Kavoussi LR, Clayman RV, Ehrlich R, Evans R, Fuchs G, Gersham A, Hulbert JC, McDougall EM, Rosenthal T, Schuessler WW, Shepard T. Complications of laparoscopic nephrectomy in 185 patients: a multi-institutional review. J Urol 1995; 154:479–483.
38. Dunn MD, Portis AJ, Shalhav Al, McDougall EM, Clayman RV. Laparoscopic versus open radical nephrectomy for renal tumors: a nine year experience. J Urol 2000; 164:1153–1160.
39. Shichman SJ, Wong JE, Sosa E, Berlin BB. Hand assisted laparoscopic radical nephrectomy and nephroureterectomy: a new standard for the 21st century. J Urol 1999; 161:23A.
40. Abbou CC, Cicco A, Gasman D, Hoznek A, Antiphon A, Chopin DK, Salomon L. Retroperitoneal laparoscopic versus open radical nephrectomy. J Urol 1999; 161:1776–1780.
41. Hsu TH, Gill IS, Matin SF, Soble JJ, Sung GT, Schweizer D, Novick AC. Radical nephrectomy and nephroureterectomy in the octogenarian and nonagenarian: comparison of laparoscopic and open approaches. Urology 1999; 53:1121–1124.
42. Ono Y, Ohshima S, Hirabayashi S, Hatano Y, Sakakibara T, Kobayashi H, Ichikawa Y. Laparoscopic nephrectomy using a retroperitoneal approach: comparison with a transabdominal approach. Int J Urol 1995; 2:12–16.

43. Winfield HN, Donovan JF, Godet AS. Human laparoscopic partial nephrectomy: case report. J Endourol 1992; 6:559.

44. Gill IS, Delworth MG, Munch LC. Laparoscopic retroperitoneal partial nephrectomy. J Urol 1994; 152:1539.

45. McDougall EM, Clayman RV, Chandhoke PS. Laparoscopic partial nephrectomy in the pig model. J Urol 1993; 149:1633–1636.

46. Gill IS, Munch LC, Clayman RV. A new renal tourniquet for open and laparoscopic partial nephrectomy. J Urol 1995; 154:1113–1116.

47. Elashry OM, Wolf JS, Rayala HJ. Recent advances in laparoscopic partial nephrectomy: comparative study of electrosurgical snare electrode and ultrasound dissection. J Endourol 1997; 11:15–22.

48. Hsu TH, Gill IS, Sung GT, Meraney AM, McMahon J, Novick AC. Laparoscopic aorto-renal bypass. J Endourol 2000; 14:123–127.

49. Kozlowski PM, Winfield HN. Laparoscopic partial nephrectomy and wedge resection. J Endourol 2000; 14:865–871.

50. Janetschek G, Daffner P, Peschel R, Bartsch G. Laparoscopic nephron sparing surgery for small renal cell carcinoma. J Urol 1998; 159:1152–1155.

51. Watanabe R, Kurumada S, Go H. Laparoscopic partial nephrectomy via the retroperitoneal approach: an animal experiment. J Urol 1997; 157:38A.

52. Hernandez AD, Smith JA, Jeppson KG. A controlled study of the argon beam coagulator for partial nephrectomy. J Urol 1990; 143:1062–1064.

53. McDougall EM, Elbahnasy AM, Clayman RV. Laparoscopic wedge resection and partial nephrectomy—the Washington University experience and review of the literature. J Soc Laparoendosc Surg 1998; 2:15–23.

54. Hozek A, Salomon L, Antiphon P, Radier C, Hafiani M, Chopin DK, Abbou CC. Partial nephrectomy with retroperitoneal laparoscopy. J Urol 1999; 162:1922–1926.

55. Rassweiler JJ, Abbou CC, Janetschek G, Jeschke K. Laparoscopic partial nephrectomy: the European experience. Urol Clin North Am 2000; 27:721–726.

56. Iverson AJ, Harmon WJ, Bishoff JT, Kavoussi LR. Laparoscopic nephron-sparing surgery for T1 solid renal masses: hemostasis and tumor control. J Urol 2000; 165S:20.

57. Desai M, Gill IS, Murphy DP, Kaouk JH, Meraney AM, Schweizer DK, Sung GT, Novick AC. Pure laparoscopic partial nephrectomy for renal tumors: duplicating open surgical principles. J Urol 2000; 165S:157.

58. Cadeddu JA, Ono Y, Clayman RV, Barrett PH, Janetschek G, Fentie DD, McDougall EM, Moore RG, Kinukawa T, Elbahnasy AM, Nelson JB, Kavoussi LR. Laparoscopic nephrectomy for renal cell cancer: evaluation of efficacy and safety: a multicenter experience. Urology 1998; 52:773–777.

59. Rafla S. Renal cell carcinoma: natural history and results of treatment. Cancer 1970; 25:26–31.

60. Finney R. An evaluation of postoperative radiotherapy in hypernephroma treatment: a clinical trial. Cancer 1973; 32:1322–1326.

61. Alter AJ, Uehling PT, Zweibel WJ. Computerized tomography of the retroperitoneum following nephrectomy. Radiology 1979; 133:663–667.

62. Sease WC, Belis JA. Computerized tomography in the early postoperative management of renal cell carcinoma. J Urol 1986; 136:792–795.

63. Saitoh H, Nakamura K. Distant metastases of renal adenocarcinoma in nephrectomized cases. J Urol 1983; 127:1092–1095.

64. Castilho LN, Fugita OEH, Mitre AI, Arap S. Port site tumor recurrences of renal cell carcinoma after videolaparoscopic radical nephrectomy. J Urol 2000; 175:519.
65. Jackman SV, Cadeddu JA, Chen RN, Micali S, Bishoff JT, Lee BR, Moore RG, Kavoussi LR. Utility of the harmonic scalpel for laparoscopic partial nephrectomy. J Endourol 1998; 12:441–444.

6

Laparoscopic Surgery of the Ureter and Bladder

Deborah Glassman

Department of Urology, Jefferson University School of Medicine, Philadelphia, Pennsylvania, USA

Steven G. Docimo

Department of Pediatric Urology, The University of Pittsburgh School of Medicine, Children's Hospital of Pittsburgh, Pittsburgh, Pennsylvania, USA

HISTORY

Laparoscopy in urology began largely as a diagnostic tool for the nonpalpable testis (1). Urological possibilities for laparoscopy became apparent when the first laparoscopic nephrectomies were performed (2). Since that time, the indications for and techniques of urologic laparoscopic surgery have expanded as rapidly as imagination and instrumentation have allowed. Laparoscopy for the ureter and bladder has been performed for extirpative procedures, but the exciting future is in reconstruction. Pediatric laparoscopic pyeloplasty was published as early as 1995 (3), but remains a procedure that is performed in only a handful of centers due to the technical complexity of suturing. The first laparoscopic bladder augmentation was performed in 1994 (4), but the technique is complicated enough so that very few have been performed, and almost all of these have been in adults (5). At about the same time, bladder autoaugmentation was performed laparoscopically (6). This is an ideal operation for adaptation to laparoscopic techniques, but its long-term outcomes have been controversial. Reconstructive procedures of the lower urinary tract can be performed in a laparoscopic-assisted manner (7). All this represents a step forward, especially for pediatric patients who require bladder augmentation and/or continent stomas. Laparoscopic-assisted reconstruction hopefully represents a way station as the techniques and instruments for complex laparoscopic procedures continue to develop.

TRANSPERITONEAL VS. RETROPERITONEAL APPROACH

Approaching the ureter and bladder, like the kidney, can be done transperitoneally or retroperitoneally. The most quoted advantage of the retroperitoneal approach is that the peritoneum is not violated. This may decrease postoperative complications such as ileus, adhesion, or hernia formation, though none of these have been demonstrated to date. The more compelling advantage of retroperitoneoscopy is easier exposure of the renal hilum in some cases. However, the transperitoneal route can be less confusing to the surgeon as it often is more familiar anatomically. It also allows more room for port placement affording a larger working space.

Transperitoneal insufflation of the abdomen is usually performed by Veress needle with percutaneous placement of the first port. The Hasson open technique can also be used to gain access to the abdomen when there is a question about adhesions or about the safety of blindly passing the trocar. A modified technique using a radially dilating trocar allows open access through a very small incision (8). The abdomen is typically insufflated to 15 mm of carbon dioxide gas. This is in contrast to retroperitoneal access, which is almost always obtained via an open technique, although in 1997, an ultrasound guided technique was described that placed a Veress needle in the retroperitoneal space prior to insufflation (9).

In 1992, Gaur described using a glove attached to a port site as a balloon to develop the retroperitoneal plane (10). Since then, several techniques have been described. Saline filled balloons were described by Rassweiler et al. (11) in 1994. This hydraulic technique was used to gain access first blindly, then it was modified to allow placement of a camera in the balloon to provide direct vision. Depending on patient size the balloon is distended between 500 and 1200 cc of saline. Several companies now manufacture balloons based on this original idea. The retroperitoneum is insufflated to 15 mm CO_2 for the placement of the remaining ports and then turned down to 10–12 mm CO_2. A retrospective comparison between retroperitoneal and transperitoneal approaches to the kidney was made by McDougall et al. (12). They found no significant differences between the two techniques but recommended that the retroperitoneal approach be reserved for the treatment of benign disease.

Gill et al., in 1995, described a double-balloon technique using a balloon filled with saline to gain initial access to the retroperitoneal space. They continued the dissection inferiorly toward the pelvis with a second, smaller balloon to mobilize the peritoneum medially. With this technique they were able to perform a nephroureterectomy down to the level of the bladder demonstrating that the retroperitoneal approach need not always be reserved for benign conditions (13).

LAPAROSCOPIC TOOLS SPECIFIC TO URETERAL SURGERY

Illuminated Stents

During laparoscopic surgery of the retroperitoneum it is important to prevent unintentional injury to the ureter and to identify it for dissection and ligation when necessary. Placement of a ureteric stent preoperatively can aid in defining the ureter. There are a number of stents that can be placed that transilluminate the ureter so that it can be identified visually, as well as tactilely. The use of these stents was first described in 1983 by Kasulke (14). Several companies manufacture illuminated stents including Storz, Cook, and Rusch (15). Storz also makes a stent to be connected to a xenon light source. The laparoscopic light source is diminished and the stent source is turned on, making the stent in the ureter visible. The greatest use for illuminated stents is for procedures in which the ureter may be inadvertently injured, such as a bowel resection or adhesiolysis. There has been little application for illuminated stents in urological laparoscopy.

Alternative Anastomotic Techniques

Laparoscopic suturing is an advanced skill requiring a steep learning curve to master. Several compounds have been studied to alleviate the need to anastomose the ureter with suture. Among these are fibrin glue, recorcin, and laser welding. Fibrin glue is a mixture of $CaCl_2$, thrombin, fibrinogen, and aprotinin. It is manufactured by Immuno, Vienna, Austria, and Tissucol, Immuno, France, and is delivered by a duploject system. Fibrin glue was first used during laparoscopic reconstruction by McKay et al. (16) in 1994. While some literature suggests that fibrin glue may be a good alternative to suturing, there is controversy about its long-term efficacy. In a porcine model the fibrin glue anastomosis was able to withstand supraphysiologic pressure and was more efficacious than other adhesive techniques (17). However, in another pig model the anastomoses broke down resulting in urinoma and death (18). At present, laparoscopic suturing remains the procedure of choice for ureteral anastomosis.

PROCEDURES

Laparoscopic Pyeloplasty

A number of minimally invasive approaches to ureteropelvic junction obstruction have been developed over the past two decades. The most commonly employed has been endopyelotomy, whether through a percutaneous antegrade approach or a ureteroscopic approach (19–21). The Accucise endopyelotomy has also been widely used, a technique in which a dilating balloon is coupled with an electrocautery cutting wire, allowing the procedure to be performed under fluoroscopic guidance (22,23). The gold standard for management of the ureteropelvic junction obstruction remains the open pyeloplasty, with a success rate very close to 100% (24). This is as opposed to success rates for endopyelotomy that achieve at best 85% (25). Laparoscopic pyeloplasty represents a natural compromise: a formal reconstruction of the ureteropelvic junction similar to open pyeloplasty, yet truly a minimally invasive approach. Unfortunately, techniques for laparoscopic suturing are still difficult enough so that laparoscopic pyeloplasty, although increasing in popularity, remains a technique performed mostly at a handful of institutions. This is especially true in pediatrics, where automatic suturing devices are not routinely applicable (26).

The potential advantages of laparoscopic pyeloplasty are similar to those for other laparoscopic procedures. These include a more rapid recovery, less postoperative pain, and a better cosmetic outcome (Fig. 6.1). In addition, however, laparoscopy might allow improved access with better visualization of crossing vessels (Fig. 6.2). The high magnification afforded by a laparoscopy is also advantageous, both in dissection and potentially in reconstruction of the ureteropelvic junction.

In experienced hands, laparoscopic pyeloplasty has been highly successful in adults, approaching or even achieving the success rates expected for open procedures (27). This experience is easily transferred to the adolescent population. In younger children, the procedure becomes more technically demanding due to smaller working spaces as well as smaller structures to be reconstructed. This is especially true in infants and young toddlers, and very few procedures have been performed or published in this age group (28).

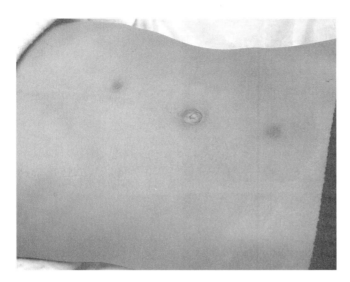

Figure 6.1 Appearance of the abdomen in a child 1 week after laparoscopic pyeloplasty, demonstrating an excellent cosmetic result.

Open pyeloplasty is almost universally performed as a retroperitoneal procedure. As in other retroperitoneal operations, this has led some to criticize the transabdominal laparoscopic approach. There is probably little disadvantage in this approach because of the documented lack of postlaparoscopic adhesion formation (29,30), but several groups have worked to develop retroperitoneal endoscopic approaches to pyeloplasty (31). The transperitoneal route allows more space for suturing, and this can be a significant factor in the younger child. For many surgeons, the transperitoneal approach may be more familiar anatomically, and therefore may be advantageous. It also may be easier to transpose the ureteropelvic junction anterior to crossing vessels via a transperitoneal approach. On the left side, a transmesenteric approach has been used by the authors, allowing reconstruction of the ureteropelvic junction without mobilizing the colon. This has some of the advantages of both approaches.

Several patterns of laparoscopic port placement have been suggested for pyeloplasty. The ergonomics of suturing must be considered when choosing port placement sites (32). The angle between the right- and left-hand instruments, as well as the camera angle, must be taken into account.

The patient should be given broad-spectrum antibiotics prior to the procedure. Consideration of bowel preparation with at least an enema the night before might be helpful, especially in left-sided procedures. Prior to the start of the operation, cystoscopy can be performed and a guide wire coiled in the renal pelvis. This is sutured to the urethral meatus and prepped into the operative field after the patient is repositioned. We start with the patient in a nearly full

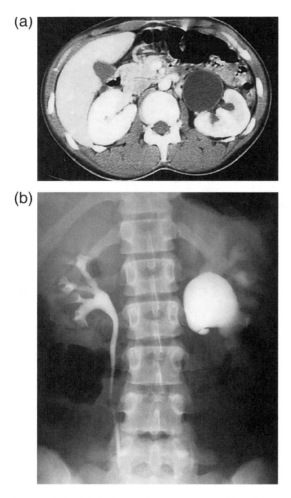

(a)

(b)

Figure 6.2 (a) CT scan demonstrates a dilated kidney consistent with ureteropelvic junction obstruction. (b) This view of an intravenous urogram reveals kinking at the Uneterophric junction typical of crossing lower pole vessels. This was confirmed at the time of laparoscopic pyeloplasty.

flank position. Initial access is obtained using an open technique in children (8), and the Veress needle technique in adults via the umbilicus (33). Initially, a midline epigastric 5 mm trocar and an ipsilateral lower-quadrant 5 mm trocar are placed. Dissection begins by either aggressively mobilizing the colon to expose the renal hilum or identifying the area of ureteropelvic junction through the colonic mesentery and creating a small window in the mesentery to expose the upper ureter.

The ureter is followed in a cephalad direction. It is important not to skeletonize the ureter in order to maintain adequate vascularity at the site of anastomosis. Dissection is continued until either the ureteropelvic junction is fully exposed or the anterior crossing vessels have been identified. Careful dissection behind crossing vessels can allow the ureteropelvic junction to be exposed inferiorly, or alternatively, the pelvis can be exposed and dissected cephalad to the crossing vessels, and the ureteropelvic junction brought above the vessels after the ureter is divided below.

A Carter–Thomason device (Close-Sure, Inlet Medical) is used to pass both ends of a stay suture in the anterior renal pelvis through the anterior abdominal wall. This is used to stabilize the pelvis before the remainder of the dissection and for the anastomosis.

When pyeloplasty is performed open, it is nearly always done in a dismembered fashion. This would suggest that laparoscopic pyeloplasty should also be done dismembered if at all possible. Because of the more difficult nature of reconstruction, other techniques have been used with success. These include the Fenger pyeloplasty, which is essentially a Heineke–Miculicz reconfiguration of the ureteropelvic junction. The Foley Y–V plasty has also been used laparoscopically with success. Most adult series of laparoscopic pyeloplasty have employed the Endostitch (US Surgical) (26). The perpendicular attachment of the suture to the needle in this device creates a traumatic needle passage that is not appropriate for pediatric reconstruction. Therefore, familiarity with laparoscopic suturing and knot tying is imperative for the performance of pediatric laparoscopic pyeloplasty. Generally, the back wall of the anastomosis is run with absorbable suture. The wire that was previously coiled in the renal pelvis is brought out through one of the laparoscopic ports, and a double-pigtail ureteral stent is passed either antegrade or retrograde and positioned in the bladder and renal pelvis. The wire is removed and the anterior wall of the anastomosis is completed. Postoperative wound drainage is generally not required if the anastomosis is stented.

The future of laparoscopic pyeloplasty almost certainly involves the use of robotic assistance. Animal studies have demonstrated the utility of robots in pyeloplasty (34), but this technology has yet to be widely applied to humans.

Large series of laparoscopic pyeloplasties in adults have demonstrated excellent outcomes (27). In children, fewer procedures have been reported. Of 18 procedures in one series, 2 required secondary laparoscopic pyeloplasty and all were eventually successful (28). Of 13 procedures performed through retroperitoneal access, 12 were successful (31). Potential complications of laparoscopic pyeloplasty include bleeding, blood transfusion, recurrent obstruction requiring endopyelotomy or reoperative pyeloplasty, bowel or other intraperitoneal injury, urinoma, and anastomotic disruption.

Laparoscopic pyeloplasty is an operation that is likely to become the standard of care over the next generation (35). Improvement in techniques and instrumentation, especially wider availability of robotic assistance, will be required for this to happen. At this time, laparoscopic pyeloplasty remains a viable alternative to open surgery, with advantages that offset the longer operating times required for this procedure.

Ureterolithotomy

Prior to the advent of endourology and percutaneous approaches to renal and ureterolithiasis, open surgery was the only option for management of symptomatic and obstructing stones. With the explosion of minimally invasive techniques for stone management traditional procedures then fell by the wayside. Open surgery was used only after other methods had failed. In 1979, laparoscopic principles were first applied to the management of these refractory cases (36). Recently, there has been a resurgence in interest in the management of these large, impacted renal pelvic or ureteral stones by laparoscopic pyelolithotomy or ureterolithotomy. Both transperitoneal and retroperitoneal approaches have been used to access the ureter.

Between 1993 and 2001 there have been seven published series, of more than eight patients, on the subject. One of the most recent, by Skrepetis et al. (37) compares open to laparoscopic transperitoneal ureterolithotomy. The advantages to laparoscopic procedures included shorter hospital stay and convalescence, lower pain medicine requirement, and fewer complications when compared to open surgery. In this series, the operating time was longer than for open surgery (85 vs. 130 min). However, the average length of operating time among all of the series is 103 min. Approaches to the ureter were both trans- and retroperitoneal according to the surgeon's preference. In general, ureteral stents were placed perioperatively and most often the ureterotomies were closed. Uniformly, closed suction drains were placed in the retroperitoneum at the conclusion of the case to drain any urine leak. In half of the studies, estimated blood loss was not recorded but the average among all of the studies was < 100 cc. Immediate postoperative complications were few among the studies, but the longest follow-up was only 6 months (38).

Ureterolysis

Extrinsic compression of the ureter may be due to a variety of etiologies. These include retroperitoneal fibrosis, malignancy, inflammatory bowel disease, and abdominal aortic aneurysms. The mainstay of therapy has been open ureterolysis. Laparoscopic ureterolysis was first reported by Kavoussi et al. (39) in 1992. The procedure is done transperitoneally. This allows for omental wrapping of the ureter or allowing an intraperitoneal course to prevent recurrence.

In a comparison of seven open to six laparoscopic ureterolysis procedures, the patients in the laparoscopic group had a shorter recovery time and less need for narcotic pain medicine. The outcome, based on IVP, was equally good for both groups (40). While this is a small study, it confirms that the laparoscopic procedure is feasible and safe. There have been several other case reports, including treatment of bilateral disease in a single setting (41).

Along the same lines, retrocaval ureter has been managed using laparoscopic techniques. There are only 10 cases reported in the literature, thus no conclusions can be drawn regarding outcomes, although this is a natural extension of laparoscopic techniques.

All of the authors used a transperitoneal approach. The peritoneum is incised and the ureter identified. It is freed distal and proximal to the retrocaval portion, which is then freed such that the ureter can be advanced either proximally or distally with gentle traction. A ureteral stent can be placed preoperatively and drawn distally after ureteral transection and readvanced into the renal pelvis prior to anastomosis. Intracorporeal suturing techniques are used to reattach the ureter.

Ureteral Reimplantation

Vesicoureteral reflux is an area in which minimally invasive approaches have long played a role. The subtrigonal injection of materials for management of reflux, which will not be covered here, is the most notable example. Laparoscopic techniques have been employed for the management of reflux in two ways: transvesical approaches and extravesical approaches.

Transvesical approaches are not strictly laparoscopic, because they do not involve entering the peritoneum. These are techniques in which laparoscopic instruments are introduced directly into the bladder in order to perform surgical manipulation. These techniques have been made possible by the availability of smaller instrumentation. The first clinically applied attempt at transvesical reflux management was an endoscopic adaptation of the Gil-Vernet operation, or trigonoplasty (42,43). This is an operation in which a horizontal incision is made from one ureteral orifice to the other, and then closed in a vertical direction incorporating the detrusor muscle (Fig. 6.3). This pulls the ureteral orifices toward the midline and enhances the fixation of the ureteral tunnel. Unfortunately, the long-term outcomes of endoscopic trigonoplasty have not been encouraging (44).

The next step in this evolution is toward transvesical ureteral reimplantation. It has been shown both experimentally (45) and clinically (44,46) that dissection of the ureters from the bladder muscle as well as reimplantation can be carried out using endoscopic techniques. It is unclear at this point whether the results of percutaneous reimplant justify the increased time required to do the procedure. With most open reimplants requiring only an overnight stay in the hospital, and with the minimal cosmetic impact of a low Pfannenstiel incision, it has been difficult to justify a procedure that takes longer and may not have as high a success rate.

The most widely applied laparoscopic technique for management of vesicoureteral reflux has been the extravesical ureteral reimplant (47,48). This

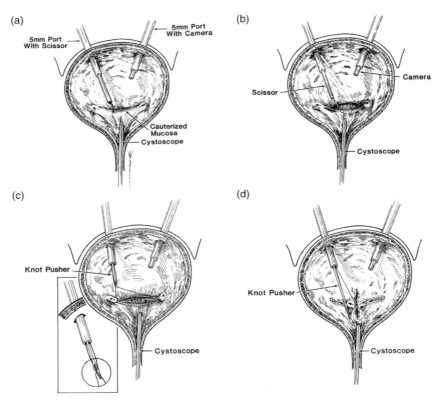

Figure 6.3 The steps of endoscopic trigonoplasty: (a, b) a longitudinal incision is made in the trigone between the ureteral orifices (c) a suture is placed, incorporating the muscle beneath the orifices. (d) the suture is tied intracorporeally to draw the orifices to the midline, enhancing the length of the ureteral tunnel. [From Cartwright et al. (43); used with permission.]

is a laparoscopic adaptation of the Lich–Gregoir technique, performed transperitoneally. This technique was first reported in minipigs in 1993 (48) and further work followed (49). The largest series from the University of Massachusetts (47). Their technique involves an incision in the peritoneum made distal and medial to the round ligament (vas deferens) isolating the ureter. After determining the most natural course of the ureter along the back wall of the bladder, a bladder stay suture is placed through the anterior abdominal wall to stabilize the bladder for further dissection. An incision is made in the detrusor to reveal the mucosa proximal to the ureteral orifice. Generally, no attempt is made to extend this beyond the ureter as is often done in the open procedure. The bladder muscle is then closed using intra-corporeal suturing techniques, incorporating the ureter in a submucosal tunnel.

Results of this single series have been impressive (47). There were 71 ureters operated on in 47 patients. There was no residual reflux or obstruction based on voiding cystourethrogram (VCUG) and ultrasound data. The initial report contains no data on the length of surgery, but currently these procedures reportedly take no longer than the open extravesical ureteral reimplant. Once again, an open operation that has little cosmetic impact and generally results in an overnight stay with nearly 100% success is not begging for an endoscopic alternative. For this reason, laparoscopic extravesical ureteral reimplantation may or may not eventually become a standard procedure.

Cystectomy

The application of laparoscopy to extirpative bladder surgery was first reported in 1992 when Parra and Bouillier (50) performed a simple cystectomy for benign disease. Indications for simple cystectomy include neurogenic bladder, pyocystis, and intractable pain from interstitial cystitis, radiation, fistula formation, or tuberculosis. With further experience, laparoscopic techniques have been applied to bladder malignancy. de Badajoz et al. (51,52) reported laparoscopic radical cystectomy in 1993.

The patient is placed in low lithotomy position and well padded. The shoulders must be monitored as steep Trendelenberg positioning is used during the procedure to keep the bowel out of the field. Four to six ports are placed in a semicircle around the bladder. The procedure is done transperitoneally to allow access to the bladder from the posterior aspect. This allows the rectum to drop down early in the procedure. In a male patient, the vasa are divided, as are the obliterated umbilical arteries. The seminal vesicles are identified and Denonvilliers' fascia is divided as well to further drop the rectum away from the bladder and prostate. The ureters are identified as they enter the bladder. This then defines the lateral pedicles, which can be divided using a laparoscopic stapler. After the posterior and lateral dissection is complete the anterior peritoneum is opened and the prevesical space enlarged. The puboprostatic ligaments and the dorsal venous complex are ligated and divided. The urethra is transected to free the specimen.

In a female patient the uterus and ovaries are delivered with the specimen as the posterior peritoneum is divided in the cul-de-sac. The laparoscopic stapler is used to divide uterine ligaments and bladder pedicles. The ureters are divided at the bladder wall as in the male. The vagina is opened and the urethra is divided. The specimen can then be delivered transvaginally, as first described by Puppo et al. (53), or through a minilaparotomy or port site extension. In a male patient, the specimen is placed in a bag and delivered through a port site extension, minilaparotomy incision or transanally (54).

Extracorporeal reconstruction and ileal loop urinary diversion can been performed through a minilaparotomy incision after laparoscopic cystectomy. However, intracorporeal urinary diversion and bladder reconstruction represent the cutting edge of laparoscopic techniques. Kozminski and Partmanian (55) first reported ileal loop creation using laparoscopic techniques in 1992. The ileal segment was isolated and the bowel was reanastomosed intracorporeally. The uretero-ileal anastomosis was performed extracorporeally through the stoma site.

The first entirely intracorporeal construction of an ileal loop was performed in a porcine model by Fergany et al. (56). Using laparoscopic staplers the ileal loop was isolated from the bowel. The bowel was then brought back into continuity. The distal end of the loop was delivered outside the body to the selected stoma site. The stoma was then matured. The ureteral anastomoses were formed using freehand suturing techniques over single J stents. Their results were promising although they experienced a significant amount of stomal stenosis at the skin level (60%). The authors attributed this to characteristics of the pig healing and not to the technique. They implied that it would not happen in a human model. In fact, when these authors then went on to perform the same operation in two people, there were no stomal complications (57).

Taking laparoscopic skills one step further this same group has gone on to perform intracorporeal creation of an orthotopic ileal neobladder (58). Moving back to the porcine model, a Studer pouch (59,60) was formed in 12 animals after cystectomy. While the ileal loop was created using stapling devices, the pouch was primarily hand sewn. Urodynamic parameters and bladder capacity were adequate. All animals had ureteral reflux. This was attributed to the inability to teach the pigs to void regularly and the need to try and catheterize them while they are distracted. This procedure will be applied to patients with low-stage disease, as the open procedure now is.

Another alternative to the Studer pouch for continent urinary diversion is the rectal sigmoid pouch. Turk et al. (54,61) have developed an intracorporeal technique to create such a Mainz II pouch. Five patients underwent the procedure. The bowel was reconfigured with hand-sewn suture lines and the ureters were stented. Although there is no long-term follow-up, the patients did well in the perioperative period. All patients were continent of stool and urine immediately postoperatively.

Laparoscopic Management of Urinary Incontinence

Stress urinary incontinence (SUI) was first managed surgically nearly a century ago (62). Since that time there have been dozens of techniques and modifications of those procedures described to treat SUI. The proliferation of techniques is a testament to the lack of long-term success of most of these bladder outlet procedures. In recent years, the colposuspension, needle urethopexy, and pubovaginal sling procedures have emerged as the techniques used most commonly in the management of SUI. The various forms of needle suspension represented minimally invasive attempts to correct stress urinary incontinence. With laparoscopy, the potential is for a more formal operation performed through a minimally invasive approach.

In 1991, Vancaillie and Schuessler (63) published the first laparoscopic colposuspension series. Multiple case reports and small series have subsequently been published. Unfortunately, there is little uniformity in the techniques to be able to make comparisons between the studies. Reported cure rates for suspensions and urethropexies, as summarized by Miklos and Kohli (64), range from 70% to 100%, with the majority greater than 80% and follow-up time ranging from 4 to 30 months. In comparison to open techniques there was early evidence that the laparoscopic urethropexy procedure may have a better outcome than similar open procedures (65). The success rate in Polascik's study was 83% for the laparoscopic procedure compared to 70% for the open technique. However, the follow-up for the open retropubic urethropexy was 15 months longer, possibly explaining the difference.

The technique of laparoscopic colposuspension involves development of the space of Retzius. The patient is placed in dorsal lithotomy or frog-leg position. A catheter allows the bladder to be drained and filled as necessary to aid in dissection and identification of the paravaginal/periurethral tissue. Insufflation with a Veress needle for a transperitoneal approach or open placement of a trocar with a dissecting balloon in the retropubic space, for an extraperitoneal approach, allows the definition of the correct plane. Three trocars, on average, are placed to provide access to the working space. Sutures are passed between the periurethral fascia and Cooper's ligament and secured. Upward pressure on the urethra and anterior vaginal wall can aid in tying the sutures. Cystoscopy may be performed to ensure that the sutures did not transgress the urethral mucosa or bladder and that ureteral obstruction has not occurred. If necessary, anterior colporraphy can also be performed laparoscopically by securing the paravaginal tissue to the pubic symphysis and ischial spines. Other than the urethral catheter, no drainage is required. An alternative to laparoscopic suturing is the use of synthetic hernia mesh to secure the periurethral/perivaginal tissue to Cooper's ligament. Using the mesh and tacking devices originally developed for inguinal hernia repair allows for shorter operating times. This makes these procedures more generally applicable, rather than limited to those with intracorporeal suturing skill (66).

Despite the initial promising results of the laparoscopic bladder neck suspension, long-term outcomes have been disappointing. McDougall et al. (67), reported that the success rate for laparoscopic colposuspension after a median of 40 months was only 50%. Most patients failed after 18–24 months. This has been reiterated in the findings of Das (68), who at 36 months had a success rate of 40% for laparoscopic suspension. These outcomes seem worse than the long-term results of open Burch colposuspension, which have been reported at 69% at 10–12 years (69).

Laparoscopic Bladder Reconstruction

Laparoscopy and minimally invasive approaches are only beginning to have an impact on bladder reconstruction. This is because of the complexity of these reconstructive procedures and the difficulty of working in the deep pelvis.

A number of advances have been made, and over the next decade, bladder reconstructive procedures will be more commonly performed laparoscopically.

The indications for bladder reconstruction are similar whether open or laparoscopic techniques are used. These include poor bladder compliance, small bladder volume, and intractable uninhibited bladder contractions. The principal of bladder reconstruction is to create a low-pressure, high-volume urinary reservoir with adequate bladder neck resistance to produce dryness. Bladder neck resistance may be achieved through division of the bladder neck, bladder neck reconstruction, bladder neck sling procedures or with the artificial urinary sphincter. Often, the urethra is not appropriate for catheterization, due to patient confinement to a wheelchair, body habitus, or a previous urethral reconstruction. In these cases, a continent catheterizable stoma can be created.

The operative steps in these procedures are the same whether they are performed in an open or a laparoscopic manner. These include access to the abdomen and pelvis, dissection of gastrointestinal segments and lysis of adhesions, selection and mobilization of tissue for bladder augmentation and tissue for stoma creation, mobilization of the bladder and bladder neck as needed, and finally, assembly of the parts into the final configuration of the bladder.

Complete laparoscopic bladder augmentation has been performed relatively rarely. The first operation was a laparoscopic gastrocystoplasty performed in 1994 (4) (Fig. 6.4). This was a successful operation, but took nearly 11 h to complete. After this case report, gastrointestinal bladder augmentation was not routinely performed for some time. During this time, laparoscopic autoaugmentation was developed. Autoaugmentation is a technique for increasing bladder capacity and compliance by dividing the bladder muscle, allowing the mucosa to act as a diverticulum (70). This procedure lends itself to a laparoscopic approach due to its relative simplicity and lack of a large anastomosis. Laparoscopic autoaugmentation was initially performed in a transperitoneal manner (71). Preperitoneal autoaugmentation has also been described and has been used with some success (6). Although autoaugmentation is suitable for selected patients with neurogenic bladder and other bladder ailments, overall long-term success has been less than optimal.

There has recently been a resurgence of interest in laparoscopic gastrointestinal bladder augmentation. Nearly all of these procedures have been performed in adults (5). The technique used most commonly involves an extracorporeal bowel anastomosis with laparoscopic bladder anastomosis. Three adult cases were recently reported, all with successful outcomes (5).

The current state-of-the-art for minimally invasive bladder reconstruction is the laparoscopic assisted reconstruction (7,72). If one looks at the steps of bladder reconstruction listed earlier, it becomes evident that the only steps that require upper abdominal access are dissection, lysis of adhesions, and selection and mobilization of gastrointestinal segments. Mobilizing the

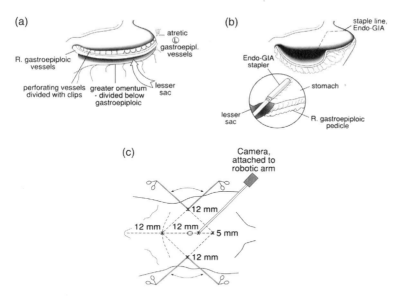

Figure 6.4 Laparoscopic stomach harvest. (a) The gastroepiploic vessels are carefully separated from the greater curve to create the pedicle. (b) Multiple firings of an endoscopic gastrointestinal stapler are used to separate the segment from the remainder of the stomach. (c) Trocar placement allows work in the upper abdomen as well as in the pelvis without duplicating the lateral ports. [from Docimo et al. (4); used with permission.]

bladder, reconstructing the bladder neck, and assembling the parts into a final reconstruction can all be accomplished through a fairly small Pfannenstiel or lower-midline incision. This is the concept behind laparoscopic-assisted reconstruction.

In most of these procedures, a continent umbilical stoma is being formed. For this reason, open access is achieved through a curvilinear lower umbilical incision that creates a posterior umbilical flap for later incorporation into the stoma (73,74). A radially dilating trocar is ideal for this form of open access (8). Trocars are then placed according to the eventually planned lower-abdominal incision. Generally, one trocar is placed along the planned incision, and a second is placed in the midepigastrium. Lysis of adhesions and mobilization of the cecum and appendix or other gastrointestinal segments are carried out. The presence of a ventriculoperitoneal shunt, common in pediatric patients requiring bladder augmentation, is not a contraindication to laparoscopy (75).

Laparoscopic mobilization of the augmentation segments can take many forms. Stomach has been mobilized on a gastroepiploic pedicle (4) (Fig. 6.4). Laparoscopic nephrectomy has been carried out with harvesting of the ureter for ureteral augmentation. The right or left colon can be mobilized, and the appendix can be harvested laparoscopically or through the open lower-abdominal incision.

Once all of the components for reconstruction easily reach a lower-abdominal incision, the reconstruction can be carried out using well-established open techniques. This might include bladder neck division or reconstruction, ureteral reimplantation, bladder augmentation, and creation of a continent stoma. The incision necessary to perform these procedures is remarkably small (Fig. 6.5).

The results of laparoscope-assisted reconstruction have been at least as good as standard open surgery. In one comparative series of continent stomas, laparoscope-assisted procedures took no longer to perform, proceeded to regular diet in less than half the time, and had a hospital stay that was 3 days less than their open counterparts. There were fewer complications in the laparoscopic-assisted group, and over the short term more revisions were required in the group undergoing standard open surgery (76). Long-term outcomes of laparoscopic-assisted reconstructions also compare very favorably to conventional techniques, with a stomal revision rate of 7.7% at nearly 3 years mean follow-up and 95% of stomas continent and functional (77).

Laparoscopic bladder reconstruction is in its infancy. Dramatic advances are likely over the next decade due to both imaginative application of current

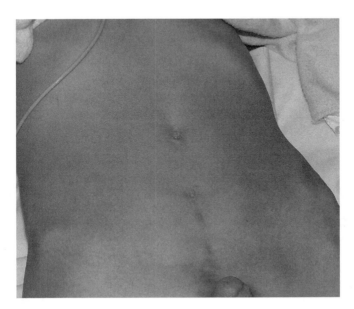

Figure 6.5 (**See color insert following page 150**) This boy with the exstrophy–epispadias complex underwent continent stoma formation and bladder neck reconstruction, and all this was accomplished through his original lower-midline incision.

technologies as well as new instrumentation and robotic support. Although experience with minimally invasive techniques for bladder reconstruction has been limited, it seems that there will be no need for large abdominal incisions for bladder reconstruction in the future.

COMPLICATIONS OF LAPAROSCOPIC BLADDER AND URETERAL SURGERY

Most of the information regarding injury to the genitourinary (GU) tract during laparoscopic surgery is from the gynecology literature. Rates of injury to the GU tract range from 0.8% to 10% (78–82). They include bladder puncture and ureteral transection or injury. When recognized intraoperatively they are often easily primarily repairable without long-term sequelae. Injection of methylene blue or indigo carmine may identify ureteral injury. A preoperatively placed ureteral stent may also help to identify an injured ureter. An inflated foley drainage bag indicates a disruption of the urinary system with extravasation of CO_2, and an injury should be sought and repaired. Similarly, inability to maintain pneumoperitoneum may indicate an injury with CO_2 leak.

Management of injury to the bladder during laparoscopy is a controversial issue. A review of the literature states that rates of bladder injury during laparoscopy range from 0.02% to 8.3%. Many urologists believe that open repair is a necessity for ensuring proper closure. However, there is a growing body of literature to support laparoscopic repair. The principles are the same for both open and laparoscopic repair.

The edges of the wound need to be debrided and then, using a stapler or hand sewing, the edges are reapproximated (83). There have also been reports of secondary healing with bladder catheter drainage. Finally, laparoscopic bladder fistula repair has been reported (84,85).

During laparoscopic ureteral and bladder procedures injuries can occur to other organs. These include trocar injuries to the bowel or blood vessels, thermal injuries secondary to laparoscopic devices, and stapler problems. In a survey of Canadian gynecologists 25% reported a trocar-related or pneumoperitoneum needle injury (86). Trauma may be minimized by establishing a full pneumoperitoneum after placement of the Veress needle, elevating the skin and fascia, using a visual obturator or an open technique to place the trocar (82).

Thermal injuries may occur with the use of cautery, laser, or ultrasonic scalpel. In an animal model, Tulikangas et al. (87) examined the effects of various energy sources on ureteral, bladder, and colonic tissue. They found that monopolar cauterization causes the largest amount of injury, particularly compared to ultrasonic scalpel. CO_2 laser showed the least depth of injury. These data corroborate a previous study by Baggish and Tucker (88). One must be aware of instrument placement at all times to minimize thermal injury and insure that the entire tip of the instrument can be visualized prior to applying thermal power.

Injuries to the colon, spleen, duodenum, and pancreas can occur during ureteral procedures. Colonic mesenteric windows may be created when dissecting the colon off of the ureter. If these are not recognized and repaired, the potential exists for internal hernia and bowel strangulation to occur.

SUMMARY

As in other areas of surgery, minimally invasive approaches to the urinary tract are early in development, but expanding rapidly. Laparoscopic pyeloplasty and laparoscopic-assisted lower-tract reconstruction are techniques with fairly clear advantages and well-established outcomes. The other procedures outlined have been used with less frequency, and their place in our armamentarium has yet to be clarified. The widespread interest in these approaches, combined with the innovation of many practitioners, will ensure a prominent role for laparoscopy and minimally invasive surgery in the future of urology.

REFERENCES

1. Cortesi N, Ferrari P, Zambarda E, Manenti A, Baldini A, Morano FP. Diagnosis of bilateral abdominal cryptorchidism by laparoscopy. Endoscopy 1976; 8:33–34.
2. Clayman RV, Kavoussi LR, Soper NJ et al. Laparoscopic nephrectomy: initial case report. J Urol 1991; 146:278–282.
3. Peters CA, Schlussel RN, Retik AB. Pediatric laparoscopic dismembered pyeloplasty. J Urol 1995; 153:1962–1965.
4. Docimo SG, Moore RG, Adams J, Kavoussi LR. Laparoscopic bladder augmentation using stomach. Urology 1995; 46:565–569.
5. Gill IS, Rackley RR, Meraney AM, Marcello PW, Sung GT. Laparoscopic enterocystoplasty. Urology 2000; 55:178–181.
6. McDougall EM, Clayman RV, Figenshau RS, Pearle MS. Laparoscopic retropubic auto-augmentation of the bladder. J Urol 1995; 153:123–126.
7. Hedican SP, Schulam PG, Docimo SG. Laparoscopic assisted reconstructive surgery. J Urol 1999; 161:267–270.
8. Cuellar D, Kavoussi PK, Baker LA, Docimo SG. Open laparoscopic access using a radially dilating trocar: experience and indications in 50 consecutive cases. J Endourol 2000; 14:755–756.
9. de Canniere L, Michel LA, Lorge F, Rosiere A, Vandenbossche P. Direct carbon dioxide insufflation of the retroperitoneum under laparoscopic control for renal and adrenal surgery. Eur J Surg 1997; 163:339–344.
10. Gaur DD. Laparoscopic operative retroperitoneoscopy: use of a new device. J Urol 1992; 148:1137–1139.
11. Rassweiler JJ, Henkel TO, Stoch C et al. Retroperitoneal laparoscopic nephrectomy and other procedures in the upper retroperitoneum using a balloon dissection technique. Eur Urol 1994; 25:229–236.
12. McDougall EM, Clayman RV, Fadden PT. Retroperitoneoscopy: the Washington University Medical School experience. Urology 1994; 43:446–452.

13. Gill IS, Munch LC, Lucas BA, Das S. Initial experience with retroperitoneoscopic nephroureterectomy: use of a double-balloon technique. Urology 1995; 46:747–750.
14. Kasulke RJ. Accurate intraoperative identification of the ureters with the use of ureteral illumination. Am Surg 1983; 49:501.
15. Teichman JM, Lackner JE, Harrison JM. Comparison of lighted ureteral catheter luminance for laparoscopy. Tech Urol 1997; 3:213–215.
16. McKay TC, Albala DM, Gehrin BE, Castelli M. Laparoscopic ureteral reanastomosis using fibrin glue. J Urol 1994; 152:1637–1640.
17. Eden CG. Alternative techniques for laparoscopic tissue anastomosis in the retroperitoneum. Endosc Surg Allied Technol 1995; 3:27–32.
18. Anidjar M, Desgrandchamps F, Martin L et al. Laparoscopic fibrin glue ureteral anastomosis: experimental study in the porcine model. J Endourol 1996; 10:51–56.
19. Clayman RV, Basler JW, Kavoussi L Picus DD. Ureteronephroscopic endopyelotomy. J Urol 1990; 144:246–251 (discussion 251–252).
20. Kavoussi LR, Meretyk S, Dierks SM et al. Endopyelotomy for secondary ureteropelvic junction obstruction in children. J Urol 1991; 145:345–349.
21. Tan HL, Najmaldin A, Webb DR. Endopyelotomy for pelvi-ureteric junction obstruction in children. Eur Urol 1993; 24:84–88.
22. Bolton DM, Bogaert GA, Mevorach RA, Kogan BA, Stoller ML. Pediatric ureteropelvic junction obstruction treated with retrograde endopyelotomy. Urology 1994; 44:609–613.
23. Kim FJ, Herrell SD, Jahoda AE, Albala DM. Complications of acucise endopyelotomy. J Endourol 1998; 12:433–436.
24. Hendren WH, Radhakrishnan J, Middleton AW Jr. Pediatric pyeloplasty. J Pediatr Surg 1980; 15:133–144.
25. Motola JA, Badlani GH, Smith AD. Results of 212 consecutive endopyelotomies: an 8-year followup. J Urol 1993; 149:453–456.
26. Adams JB, Schulam PG, Moore RG, Partin AW, Kavoussi LR. New laparoscopic suturing device: initial clinical experience. Urology 1995; 46:242–245.
27. Jarrett T, Chan D, Charambura T, Fugita O, Kavoussi L. Laparoscopic pyeloplasty: the first 100 cases. J Urol 2002; 167:1253–1256.
28. Tan HL. Laparoscopic Anderson-Hynes dismembered pyeloplasty in children. J Urol 1999; 162:1045–1047 (discussion 1048).
29. Pattaras J, Moore R, Landman J et al. Incidence of postoperative adhesion formation after transperitoneal genitourinary laparoscopic surgery. Urology 2002; 59:37–41.
30. Moore RG, Kavoussi LR, Bloom DA, Bogaert GA, Jordon GH, Kogan BA. Postoperative adhesion formation after urological laparoscopy in the pediatric population. J Urol 1995; 153:792–795.
31. Yeung C, Tam Y, Sihoe J, Lee K, Liu K. Retroperitoneoscopic dismembered pyeloplasty for pelvi-ureteric junction obstruction in infants and children. BJU Int 2001; 87:509–513.
32. Frede T, Stock C, Rassweiler J, Alken P. Retroperitoneoscopic and laparoscopic suturing: tips and strategies for improving efficiency. J Endourol 2000; 14:905–913.
33. Veress J. Neus instrument zur ausfuhrung von brust-oder bachpunktionen und pneumthorax be-handlung. Dtsch Med Wochenschr 1938; 64:1480.
34. Sung G, Gill I, Hsu T. Robotic-assisted laparoscopic pyeloplasty: a pilot study. Urology 1999; 53:1099–1103.

35. Docimo SG, Kavoussi LR. The role of endourological techniques in the treatment of the pediatric ureteropelvic junction. J Urol 1997; 158:1538.
36. Wickham J. The surgical treatment of urolithiasis. In: Wickham J, ed. Urinary Calculus Disease. New York: Churchill Livingstone, 1979:183–186.
37. Skrepetis K, Doumas K, Siafakas I, Lykourinas M. Laparoscopic versus open ureterolithotomy. A comparative study. Eur Urol 2001; 40:32–36 (discussion 37).
38. Bellman GC, Smith AD. Special considerations in the technique of laparoscopic ureterolithotomy. J Urol 1994; 151:146–149.
39. Kavoussi LR, Clayman RV, Brunt LM, Soper NJ. Laparoscopic ureterolysis. J Urol 1992; 147:426–429.
40. Elashry OM, Nakada SY, Wolf JS Jr, Figenshau RS, McDougall EM, Clayman RV. Ureterolysis for extrinsic ureteral obstruction: a comparison of laparoscopic and open surgical techniques. J Urol 1996; 156:1403–1410.
41. Mattelaer P, Boeckmann W, Brauers A, Wolff JM, Jakse G. Laparoscopic ureterolysis in retroperitoneal fibrosis. Acta Urol Belg 1996; 64:15–18.
42. Okamura K, Ono Y, Yamada Y et al. Endoscopic trigonoplasty for primary vesicoureteric. Br J Urol 1995; 75:390–394.
43. Cartwright PC, Snow BW, Mansfield JC, Hamilton BD. Percutaneous endoscopic trigonoplasty: a minimally invasive approach to correct vesicoureteral reflux. J Urol 1996; 156:661–664.
44. Gatti JM, Cartwright PC, Hamilton BD, Snow BW. Percutaneous endoscopic trigonoplasty in children: long-term outcomes and modifications in technique. J Endourol 1999; 13:581–584.
45. Lakshmanan Y, Mathews RI, Cadeddu JA et al. Feasibility of total intravesical endoscopic surgery using mini-instruments in a porcine model. J Endourol 1999; 13:41–45.
46. Gill IS, Ponsky LE, Desai M, Kay R, Ross JH. Laparoscopic cross-trigonal Cohen ureteroneocystostomy: novel technique. J Urol 2001; 166:1811–1814.
47. Lakshamanan Y, Fung LC. Laparoscopic extravesicular ureteral re-implantation for vesicoureteral reflux: recent technical advances. J Endourol 2000; 14:589–593.
48. Atala A, Kavoussi LR, Goldstein DS, Retik AB, Peters CA. Laparoscopic correction of vesicoureteral reflux. J Urol 1993; 150:748–751.
49. Reddy PK, Evans RM. Laparoscopic ureteroneocystostomy. J Urol 1994; 152:2057–2059.
50. Parra RO, Boullier JA. Endocavitary (laparoscopic) bladder surgery. Semin Urol 1992; 10:213–221.
51. Sanchez de Badajoz E, del Rosal Samaniego JM, Gomez Gamez A, Burgos Rodriguez R, Vara Thorbeck C. Laparoscopic ileal conduit. Arch Esp Urol 1992; 45:761–764. (In Spanish.)
52. Sanchez de Badajoz E, Gallego Perales JL, Reche Rosado A, Gutierrez de la Cruz JM, Jimenez Garrido A. Radical cystectomy and laparoscopic ileal conduit. Arch Esp Urol 1993; 46:621–624. (In Spanish.)
53. Puppo P, Perachino M, Ricciotti G, Bozzo W, Gallucci M, Carmignani G. Laparoscopically assisted transvaginal radical cystectomy. Eur Urol 1995; 27:80–84.
54. Turk I, Deger S, Winkelmann B, Schonberger B, Loening SA. Laparoscopic radical cystectomy with continent urinary diversion (rectal sigmoid pouch) performed completely intracorporeally: the initial 5 cases. J Urol 2001; 165:1863–1866.

55. Kozminski M, Partmanian K. Case report of laparoscopic ileal loop conduit. J Endourol 1992; 6:147–150.
56. Fergany AF, Gill IS, Kaouk JH, Meraney AM, Hafez KS, Sung GT. Laparoscopic intracorporeally constructed ileal conduit after porcine cystoprostatectomy. J Urol 2001; 166:285–288.
57. Gill IS, Fergany A, Klein EA et al. Laparoscopic radical cystoprostatectomy with ileal conduit performed completely intracorporeally: the initial 2 cases. Urology 2000; 56:26–29 (discussion 29–30).
58. Kaouk JH, Gill IS, Desai MM et al. Laparoscopic orthotopic ileal neobladder. J Endourol 2001; 15:131–142.
59. Studer UE, Casanova GA, Zingg EJ. Bladder substitution with an ileal low-pressure reservoir. Eur Urol 1988; 14:36–40.
60. Studer UE. Bladder substitution with an ileal low-pressure reservoir. Prog Clin Biol Res 1989; 303:803–809.
61. Turk I, Deger S, Winkelmann B, Baumgart E, Loening SA. Complete laparoscopic approach for radical cystectomy and continent urinary diversion (sigma rectum pouch). Tech Urol 2001; 7:2–6.
62. Goebell R. Zur Operativen Beseiligung der Angeharene Incontinentia Vesicae. Agynak Urol 1910; 2:187.
63. Vancaillie TG, Schuessler W. Laparoscopic bladderneck suspension. J Laparoendosc Surg 1991; 1:169–173.
64. Miklos JR, Kohli N. Laparoscopic paravaginal repair plus burch colposuspension: review and descriptive technique. Urology 2000; 56:64–69.
65. Polascik TJ, Moore RG, Rosenberg MT, Kavoussi LR. Comparison of laparoscopic and open retropubic urethropexy for treatment of stress urinary incontinence. Urology 1995; 45:647–652.
66. Ou CS, Presthus J, Beadle E. Laparoscopic bladder neck suspension using hernia mesh and surgical staples. J Laparoendosc Surg 1993; 3:563–566.
67. McDougall EM, Heidorn CA, Portis AJ, Klutke CG. Laparoscopic bladder neck suspension fails the test of time. J Urol 1999; 162:2078–2081.
68. Das S. Comparative outcome analysis of laparoscopic colposuspension, abdominal colposuspension and vaginal needle suspension for female urinary incontinence. J Urol 1998; 160:368–371.
69. Alcalay M, Monga A, Stanton SL. Burch colposuspension: a 10–20 year follow up. Br J Obstet Gynaecol 1995; 102:740–745 (Erratum appears in Br J Obstet Gynaecol 1996;103(3):290).
70. Snow BW, Cartwright PC. Autoaugmentation of the bladder. Contemp Urol 1992; 4:41–51.
71. Braren V, Bishop MR. Laparoscopic bladder autoaugmentation in children. Urol Clin North Am 1998; 25:533–540.
72. Jordan GH, Winslow BH. Laparoscopically assisted continent catheterizable cutaneous appendicovesicostomy. J Endourol 1993; 7:517–520.
73. Ben-Chaim J, Rodriguez R, Docimo SG. Concealed umbilical stoma: description of a modified technique. J Urol 1995; 154:1169–70.
74. Glassman DT, Docimo SG. Concealed umbilical stoma: long-term evaluation of stomal stenosis. J Urol 2001; 166:1028–1030.
75. Jackman S, Weingart J, Kinsman S, Docimo S. Laparoscopic surgery in patients with ventriculoperitoneal shunts: safety and monitoring. J Urol 2000; 164:1352–1354.

76. Cadeddu JA, Docimo SG. Laparoscopic-assisted continent stoma procedures: our new standard. Urology 1999; 54:909–912.

77. Chung SY, Meldrum K, Docimo SG. Laparoscopic assisted reconstructive surgery: a 7-year experience. J Urol 2004; 171:372–375.

78. Wang PH, Lee WL, Yuan CC et al. Major complications of operative and diagnostic laparoscopy for gynecologic disease. J Am Assoc Gynecol Laparosc 2001; 8:68–73.

79. Saidi MH, Sarosdy MF, Hollimon PW, Sadler RK. Intestinal obstruction and bilateral ureteral injuries after laparoscopic oophorectomy in a patient with severe endometriosis. J Am Assoc Gynecol Laparosc 1995; 2:355–358.

80. Saidi MH, Sadler RK, Vancaillie TG, Akright BD, Farhart SA, White AJ. Diagnosis and management of serious urinary complications after major operative laparoscopy. Obstet Gynecol 1996; 87:272–276.

81. Ostrzenski A, Ostrzenska KM. Bladder injury during laparoscopic surgery. Obstet Gynecol Surv 1998; 53:175–180.

82. Hasson HM, Parker WH. Prevention and management of urinary tract injury in laparoscopic surgery. J Am Assoc Gynecol Laparosc 1998; 5:99–114.

83. Taskin O, Wheeler JM. Laparoscopic repair of bladder injury and laceration. J Am Assoc Gynecol Laparosc 1995; 2:227–229.

84. Hemal AK, Kumar R, Nabi G. Post-cesarean cervicovesical fistula: technique of laparoscopic repair. J Urol 2001; 165:1167–1168.

85. Champault G, Riskalla H, Rizk N, Tchala K. Laparoscopic resection of a bladder diverticulum. Prog Urol 1997; 7:643–646. (In French.)

86. Yuzpe AA. Pneumoperitoneum needle and trocar injuries in laparoscopy. A survey onpossible contributing factors and prevention. J Reprod Med 1990; 35:485–490.

87. Tulikangas PK, Beesley S, Boparai N, Falcone T. Assessment of laparoscopic injuries by three methods. Fertil Steril 2001; 76:817–819.

88. Baggish MS, Tucker RD. Tissue actions of bipolar scissors compared with monopolar devices. Fertil Steril 1995; 63:422–426.

7

Laparoscopic Surgery of the Testis and Ovary

Paul K. Pietrow

Division of Pediatric Urology, Vanderbilt Children's Hospital, Nashville, Tennessee, USA

John W. Brock III

Vanderbilt University Medical Center, Nashville, Tennessee, USA

TESTIS

Introduction

Cryptorchidism affects ~0.8% of all males, with rates approaching 3% in neonates. Premature infants are noted to have a higher incidence of undescended testes, although this approaches that of full-term infants as they catch up with their counterparts in age. Nearly one in five of all these children will have an intra-abdominal testis, while an additional cohort of patients will have a poorly localized gonad within the inguinal canal. Surgical management of cryptorchidism has been advocated for several reasons. (i) Scrotal placement of the testis allows for easier monitoring and self-examination of the gonad to detect solid masses, since these testes carry a significant increased risk of malignancy (1). (ii) Various authors have found that these testes appear to be histologically normal appearing prior to age 1 (2). Early orchidopexy may therefore avert or ameliorate the decreased fertility that has been associated with this anomaly. (iii) The improved cosmetic appeal of a more "normal" appearing scrotum cannot be underestimated for the psyche of young males.

The application of laparoscopic surgery has been one of the greatest technical advances in the management of nonpalpable testes. Indeed, the use of the laparoscope has allowed pediatric urologists to correctly diagnose the existence and location of undescended testes in nearly all cases, with minimal morbidity to the patient. As such, this instrument has clearly supplanted other diagnostic modalities such as ultrasonography, magnetic resonance imaging, venography, or computed tomography. More importantly, correctly performed laparoscopy can replace fruitless and potentially difficult groin and retroperitoneal explorations in those patients with questionably palpated testes. Finally, laparoscopic techniques may be applied to not only diagnostic, but also therapeutic management of undescended testes.

Technique

As noted above, up to 3% of all full-term infants have an undescended testis at birth, although nearly two-thirds of these will have resolution of this process within the first 3–6 months of life. We therefore routinely wait to perform surgical correction and/or exploration until after this point. Patients' families are fully counseled regarding potential outcomes and complications. More specifically, it is explained that the operation may result in the diagnosis of a nonexistent testis, a nonsalvageable testis, or an existing inguinal or intra-abdominal testis that may require more than one operation to complete a successful orchidopexy. It is further explained that laparoscopic findings may warrant further inguinal exploration to search for dysplastic testis remnants.

After obtaining informed consent, the patient is induced under general anesthesia. At this point the patient is placed on a rolled towel at the level of his sacrum. The legs are allowed to fall apart and a careful physical examination of the affected inguinal canal and scrotum is undertaken. If a testis or nubbin of tissue is palpated, then the laparoscopic portion of the case is abandoned and inguinal exploration is begun. If careful palpation fails to reveal a testis, then the patients' entire abdomen and genitalia are prepped and draped in usual sterile fashion. Patient, physician, and equipment placement is illustrated in Fig. 7.1.

The case is begun with the placement of a small, 3 mm InterDyne trocar at the level of the umbilicus. An open technique is almost always employed because

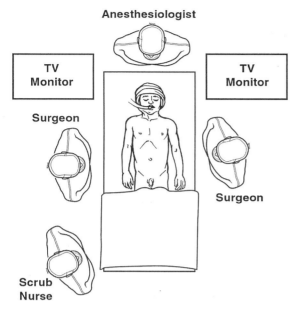

Figure 7.1   Schematic diagram of patient, physician, and monitor position during laparoscopic orchidopexy.

the loose peritoneal attachments in young children may make a closed technique (e.g., Veress needle) more dangerous. A small incision is therefore made at the inferior aspect of the umbilicus (figure) and is carried down to the level of the fascia with blunt dissection. The fascia is then incised, the rectus bellies separated, and the posterior fascia incised. Preperitoneal fat is swept aside and the peritoneum is identified and elevated. This is then divided with Metzenbaum scissors. Under direct visualization, the trocar is passed into the peritoneal cavity and secured to the abdominal fascia with synthetic absorbable sutures, which may be used later to close the fascial incision. The peritoneal cavity is then insufflated with CO_2 gas to a maximum working pressure of $12-15$ mmHg. Typical pneumoperitoneum volumes in young children average $1.0-1.5$ L.

With access obtained, a $0°$ or $30°$ laparoscope is passed via the trocar and the abdomen is inspected, beginning with those regions susceptible to trauma from the initial cutdown. The affected side is then examined for the presence and location of a testis, as well as the presence or absence of the spermatic vessels and vas deferens. The internal ring is also inspected for the presence of a gubernaculum and for patency. Typical findings at the time of laparoscopy are presented in Table 7.1.

One common scenario includes a closed internal ring with blind-ending vessels and vas as they approach the outlet (Fig. 7.2). This discovery implies

Table 7.1   Potential Laparoscopic Findings During Surgery for Nonpalpable Testis

1. Vas and spermatic vessels entering internal inguinal ring
2. Peeping testis (testis residing at internal ring)
3. Intra-abdominal testis (may require mobilization of bowel to locate gonad)
4. Blind-ending vas and vessels (vanishing testis, prenatal torsion, developmental failure)

developmental failure of the affected gonad and/or prenatal or neonatal torsion of an undescended testis. Assuming that an inguinal hernia or an open internal ring is not discovered at the time of laparoscopy, the pneumoperitoneum is released and the anterior fascial incision is closed with interrupted stitches of a synthetic absorbable suture.

If the vas deferens and spermatic vessels are seen coursing through the internal ring and the testis is not visible as a "peeping" testis, then the pneumoperitoneum is released, the access incision is closed, and inguinal exploration is performed. Small, dysplastic nubbins of tissue have been found at the time of exploration and have generally been excised. Pathologic evaluation almost always confirms a burned out testis laden with hemosiderin deposits, implying that the testis did develop but likely suffered from a prenatal torsion. The precise malignant potential of these

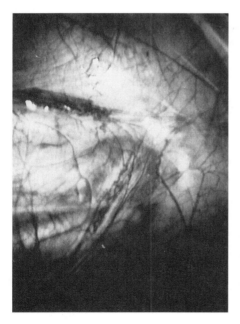

Figure 7.2   Blind-ending vas and spermatic vessels as they approach the internal ring. This is indicative of developmental failure of the gonad.

remnants is not known, but they certainly do present a theoretical risk in light of the increased incidence of germ cell tumors in these gonads.

A peeping testis is commonly found at the time of laparoscopic exploration for nonpalpable testis (Fig. 7.3). These gonads often lie within the internal ring or are able to be gently mobilized into the internal ring prior to dissection. They are not truly intra-abdominal, consequently enjoy a higher success rate with orchidopexy, and are frequently managed with a one-stage operation. Truly intra-abdominal testes are found anywhere along the course of the normal path of descent. Various maneuvers may be undertaken with the operating table to attempt to drop the bowel off of the posterior body wall. If the testis is still unable to be visualized, then the colon may sometimes be reflected to allow visualization as high as the ipsilateral kidney.

At this point it is necessary to add an additional 3 mm trocars for the passage of grasping instruments and electrocautery dissectors. At least one port will need to be of 5 mm size if a clip applier is used to perform the first stage of a two-stage Fowler–Stephens technique. All trocars should be passed under direct laparoscopic vision after transilluminating the abdominal wall to identify vessels. Two working ports are usually added on the contralateral side of the affected testis (Fig. 7.4). One port is commonly at the level of the umbilicus in the midaxillary line while the second is in the same line but lower in the abdomen. It is important to place the ports with enough space to allow the creation of traction and countertraction when performing the dissection. It is also helpful to keep these instruments in the same line of vision as the laparoscope to keep the surgeon or the camera driver from having to work "backward" from the camera.

With the working trocars in place, grasping instruments are passed through the caudad-most port, the testis is grasped and pulled toward its ipsilateral

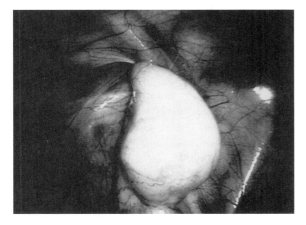

Figure 7.3 Peeping testis. Highly mobile testis found just at the entrance of the internal ring.

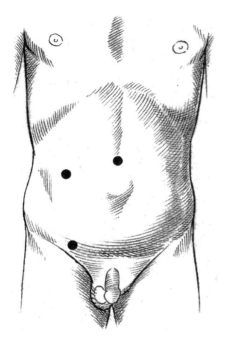

Figure 7.4   Diagram of laparoscopic port placement during orchidopexy.

internal ring. This maneuver helps determine the amount of tension on the vessels and can help predict whether a one- or two-stage procedure may be necessary.

Regardless of classification, the next step in this procedure is to begin mobilization of the spermatic vessels. The testis is therefore grasped with the caudad hand while a hook electrode or "hot" scissors are used to incise the peritoneum both laterally and medially to the spermatic vessels. The dissection is carried to the level of the kidney, taking care not to injure the spermatic vessels as the dissection proceeds cephalad.

With the gonad adequately mobilized, it is pulled toward the contralateral inguinal ring. It is widely accepted that testes with this much laxity have an excellent chance of reaching up to their ipsilateral scrotum. It is important to note that the ipsilateral vas and its attendant peritoneum have not been mobilized at this point. This could allow us to proceed to ligation of the spermatic vessels if necessary for a Fowler–Stephens type operation.

Peeping testes occasionally require vessel ligation at this point, but are still commonly managed with a one-stage procedure. If this is the case, the scrotum is then prepared by creating a dartos pouch. A transverse incision is made in the anterior surface of the scrotum and the skin is undermined with fine scissors or hemostat. When this is completed, a Kelly clamp or trocar is passed through the scrotal incision and into the abdominal compartment under direct laparoscopic vision. Care is taken to pass the clamp medial to the epigastric vessels, in essence performing a Prentiss maneuver. The testis is gently grasped with a clamp and teased through the abdominal wall into the dartos pouch. We routinely anchor the testis to the dartos tissue using synthetic absorbable sutures or a long-lasting monofilament, such as PDS. Each testis is secured with three sutures, taking care to pass the taper needle superficially through the tunica of the testis. The spermatic cord is then carefully inspected to ascertain that no twisting has occurred.

Truly intra-abdominal testes have largely required a two-stage Fowler–Stephens operation at our institution. If the cord seems short even after adequate and aggressive mobilization, then the vessels are clipped with an endoscopic clip applier and the testis is left in place in the abdominal cavity. We have routinely waited 2–3 months to allow the vasal vessels to hypertrophy prior to performing the second stage of the operation. At this point, laparoscopy can again be employed to fully divide the spermatic vessels and to mobilize the vasal pedical with a wide patch of peritoneum. The creation of the dartos pocket and the passage and securing of the testis within the scrotum are performed as described above.

We have at times treated obviously high intra-abdominal testes with primary vessel ablation with a KTP laser passed via a spinal needle through the abdominal wall (Fig. 7.5). Use of this laser without initial mobilization of the vessels allows the first stage to be performed rather expediently without the added time of multiple port placements. This technique, therefore, requires only the initial cut-down port as well as a simple puncture wound to complete

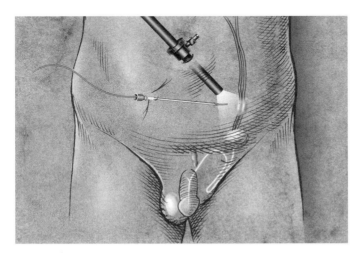

Figure 7.5 KTP laser is passed through a spinal needle to ablate the spermatic vessels during the first stage of a Fowler–Stevens orchidopexy.

the first stage. The second half of the operation is performed as described earlier for a one-stage procedure.

RESULTS

It is clear that laparoscopy has altered the approach to the nonpalpable testis. Previous studies have shown that a laparoscopic search for a hidden testis can provide accurate localization in nearly 100% of all cases (3–6). Indeed, many feel that this is the test and procedure of choice for the localization and diagnosis of a nonpalpable testis. Treatment of these gonads is also improved by the use of laparoscopic techniques. Multiple authors have reported very strong success rates with both single- and two-stage techniques.

Lindgren et al. (7, 8) have reported in two separate reports success rates of 89–100% for the treatment of intra-abdominal testes. The highest rates of success in their series were in children who had undergone no previous surgery, with several cases of atrophy in the previously operated children. Bloom reported in 1991 a series of two-stage Fowler–Stephens orchidopexies using a laparoscopic clip-applier for the first stage. He was able to achieve a satisfactory scrotal location for these intra-abdominal testes in 84% of the cases (9). Both Kaplan and Shaneberg (10) and Miller and Brock (11) have reported >90% overall success with a two-stage procedure using the KTP laser for ablation of the spermatic vessels in the first stage. More recently, Docimo (12) and others reported their data on laparoscopic orchidopexy and reported success rates of 97%, 74%, and 88% for laparoscopic orchidopexy with intact vessels, single-stage Fowler–Stephens procedures, and staged Fowler–Stephens procedures, respectively.

More recent authors have focused on the delivery of intra-abdominal testes without the need for spermatic vessel division using a wide peritoneal mobilization and gubernaculum division (13). While these results are intriguing they will need to be borne out in other institutions.

Finally, advances in instrument technology are now allowing surgeons to perform this procedure with increasingly smaller instruments. Needlescopic techniques utilizing 2 mm instruments have been described and used successfully from multiple institutions (14–16). These instruments can maintain visualization while minimizing scarring and even eliminate the need for fascial closure at the end of the procedure.

Complications

Complications from laparoscopic orchidopexy are not dissimilar from those from open procedures. Testis atrophy, failure to achieve a dependent scrotal location, and even the need for orchiectomy have been described. While the recovery from a laparoscopic search for a nonpalpable testis is quicker than an open approach, laparoscopy does offer its own set of pitfalls. There are numerous reports in the pediatric and adult literature on complications from Veress needle access to the peritoneum. Injury to the bowel, bladder, liver, spleen, and even the great vessels has been reported.

In addition, inadvertent cautery injury to intra-abdominal contents has been described from faulty grounding of laparoscopic instruments. Port sites larger than 3–4 mm are generally closed at the fascial level to prevent possible bowel herniation.

Finally, the effects of the pneumoperitoneum itself cause various physiologic changes that alter the anesthetic management of these children. It is very important to have a pediatric anesthesiologist who is experienced in the alterations of venous return and the effects of the hypercarbia from absorbed CO_2. Knowledge of these effects can prevent serious intraoperative collapse in the poorly managed patient.

OVARY

Introduction

Pediatric urologists are frequently called upon to manage both the urinary as well as the genital symptoms and diseases of young girls prior to puberty. The treatment of ovarian torsion, ovarian cysts, and ovarian teratoma and even the management of dysgenetic gonads have been described with laparoscopic techniques (17–19).

As with nonpalpable testes, some of the benefits of a laparoscopic technique in young females lie in its diagnostic capabilities coupled with the potential for therapeutic intervention. Ovarian cysts may be recognized prenatally and may present a diagnostic challenge (Fig. 7.6). Most cysts are the result of maternal

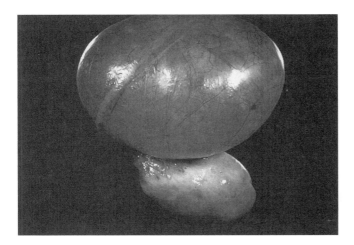

Figure 7.6   Ovarian cysts may be quite large and may present a diagnostic challenge.

hormonal stimulation and an initial rise in luteinizing and follicle-stimulating hormones. While data suggest that cysts <5 cm in size have an excellent chance of resolving within 6 months and of involving a benign process, the management of cysts larger than 5 cm can be a dilemma. There are reports that neonatal ovarian cysts larger than this cut-off may suffer from an increased risk of ovarian torsion (20) (Fig. 7.7). In addition, complex neonatal ovarian cysts may represent previous torsion or possible tumor, such as teratoma. As such, laparoscopy can clearly allow for clarification of the diagnosis as well as for surgical excision of any suspicious tissue. This technique, then, also allows the surgeon to minimize morbidity and to avoid the risks of a laparotomy in a newborn. As in torsion of the testis, one could imagine that early excision of a dead, torsed ovary may prevent potential autoimmune effects from affecting the normal, contralateral ovary.

In addition to treating neonatal ovarian torsion, laparoscopic management of torsion and even intermittent ovarian torsion in pre and postpubertal children has been described with successful outcomes (21). Ovarian torsion in this age group frequently presents as vague, but intense, lower-abdominal pain, often with an acute presentation. As expected, the differential diagnosis is quite long and can include appendicitis, ovarian torsion, ruptured ovarian cyst, ectopic pregnancy or pelvic inflammatory disease in those children who are sexually active, endometriosis, painful menses, cystitis, irritable bowels syndrome, inflammatory bowel disease, and even significant constipation. Laparoscopy may be employed as a diagnostic and therapeutic measure if the history, physical examination, laboratory, and radiologic work-up are inconclusive or suggest urgent intraabdominal pathology.

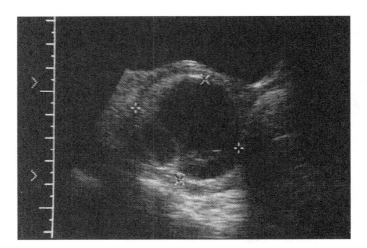

Figure 7.7 Ultrasound image of a multilocular cystic ovary found to be an ovarian torsion at the time of operation.

Ovarian teratoma is often a silent disorder and is diagnosed during evaluation for vague abdominal symptoms or during evaluation of a different process. Ultrasound imaging typically reveals a heterogenous cystic complex, often with intense echogenic regions representing cartilage or bone formation. All such lesions harbor potential malignant components and require radiologic and serologic evaluation to assess for metastases or elevations in LDH, alpha feto-protein or beta-hCG (human chorionic gonadotropin). Advanced cases of metastatic disease or peritoneal seeding after laparoscopy from lesions harboring occult malignancy have been described in women (22). Therefore, care should be taken during laparoscopic management of potential teratomas in children to avoid spillage of cyst contents. Even with such a risk, laparoscopy provides excellent visualization and the opportunity to minimize morbidity during excision of these lesions.

Various intersex disorders are associated with an increased risk of the development of malignancy within a dysgenetic gonad. This is true for pure gonadal dysgenesis, mixed gonadal dysgenesis, and even in the gonads of children with testicular feminization. Laparoscopy can provide the surgeon and patient with a minimally invasive access to the peritoneum and to the gonads of these children. Such organs can then be prophylactically excised early in life to avoid the risk of the development of a malignancy and the threat of eventual metastasis. Caution should be advised that not all such gonads will lie in a truly intraperitoneal location. Indeed, the gonads of children with testicular feminization syndrome are frequently found during the repair of supposed female inguinal hernias. However, laparoscopy can still be helpful if the diagnosis is already made and the gonads are not palpable in the inguinal canal. In this case, the procedure is carried out much like the search for a nonpalpable undescended testis.

Techniques

Laparoscopic surgery in the young female is very similar to that described for nonpalpable testes. The parents of the patient should be well informed of the risks of surgery, the potential for inadvertent injury during the initial access to the peritoneal cavity, as well as the potential for conversion to open surgery.

We recommend that the initial access port should be obtained via an open cut-down technique to avoid potential injury from the Verress needle and the initial trocar. With the trocar in position and anchored with preplaced fascial sutures, the laparoscope is passed into the abdominal cavity and a scan of the underlying tissues is performed to search for inadvertent injury. The surgeon's attention is then turned to investigating the pathology in question within the pelvis or abdominal cavity. Additional ports may be placed under direct visualization to allow for the passage of retractors or dissecting scissors, which may be necessary to sweep the overlying bowel out of the pelvis. Trendelenburg position may also be utilized to allow the bowel to fall back into the abdominal cavity.

Once adequate exposure has been achieved, attention can be turned to repairing or excising whatever pathology may be encountered. It should be noted that reports of abdominal wall/trocar seeding have surfaced following resection of ovaries bearing carcinoma and even teratoma (dermoid cysts). Ovaries that are suspected of harboring such pathology should probably be extracted via an endocatch bag or an impervious Lap-Sac (Applied Medical, Laguna Hills, CA) and an enlarged port site. Again, port sites larger than 4 mm are usually closed at the fascial level to avoid the risk of bowel herniation.

REFERENCES

1. United Kingdom Testicular Cancer Study Group. Aetiology of testicular cancer: association with congenital abnormalities, age at puberty, infertility and exercise. Br Med J 1994; 308:1393–1399.
2. Lugg JA, Penson DF, Sadegh F, Pietrie B, Freedman AL, Gonzalez-Cadavid NF, Rajfer J. Early orchidopexy versus histologic changes in cryptorchid testes [abstr 27]. J Urol 1995; 153:235a.
3. Brock JW III, Holcomb GW III, Morgan W III. The use of laparoscopy in the management of undescended testis. J Laparoendosc Surg 1996; 6(Suppl 1):535–539.
4. Holcomb GW III, Brock JW III, Neblett WW III, Pietsch JB, Morgan WM III. Laparoscopy for the nonpalpable testis. Am Surg 1994; 60:143–147.
5. Moore RG, Peters CA, Bauer SB, Mandell J, Retik AB. Laparoscopic evaluation of the impalpable testis: a prospective assessment of accuracy. J Urol 1994; 151:728–731.
6. Humphrey GM, Najmaldin AS, Thomas DF. Laparoscopy in the management of the impalpable testis. Br J Surg 1998; 85:983–985.
7. Lindgren BW, France I, Blick S, Levitt SB, Brock WA, Palmer LS, Friedman SC, Reda EF. Laparoscopic Fowler-Stephens orchidopexy for the high abdominal testis. J Urol 1999; 162(3 Pt 2):990–994.
8. Lindgren BW, Darby EC, Faiella L, Brock WA, Reda EF, Levitt SB, Franco I. Laparoscopic orchidopexy: procedure of choice for the nonpalpable testis? J Urol 1998; 159:2132–2135.
9. Bloom DA. Two step orchidopexy with pelvioscopic clip ligation of the spermatic vessels. J Urol 1991; 135:1030–1033.
10. Kaplan GW, Shaneberg A. Laser Photocoagulation of Spermatic Vessels as an Adjunct to Staged Fowler-Stephens Orchidopexy. Washington, DC: American Academy of Pediatrics, 1993.
11. Miller DA, Brock JW III. Laparoscopic KTP Laser Photocoagulation of the Testicular Vessels in First Stage Orchidopexy. New Orleans: American Academy of Pediatrics, 1997.
12. Docimo SG. Editorial. J Endourol 2001; 15:255–256.
13. Esposito C, Vallone G, Settimi A, Gonzalez Sabin MA, Amici G, Cusano T. Laparoscopic orchidopexy without division of the spermatic vessels: can it be considered the procedure of choice in intraabdominal testis? Surg Endosc 2000; 14:658–660.
14. Gill IS, Ross JH, Sung GT, Kay R. Needlescopic surgery for cryptorchidism: the initial series. J Pediatr Surg 2000; 35:1426–1430.

15. Ferrer FA, Caddedu JA, Schulam P, Mathews R, Docimo SG. Orchidopexy using 2 mm laparoscopic instruments. 2. Techniques for delivering the testis into the scrotum. J Urol 2000; 164:160–161.
16. Ilumke U, Siemer S, Bonnet L, Ziegler M. Pediatric laparoscopy for nonpalpable testis with new miniaturized instruments. J Endourol 1998; 12:445–450.
17. Decker PA, Chammas J, Sato TT. Laparoscopic diagnosis and management of ovarian torsion in the newborn. J Soc Laparoendosc Surg 1999; 3:141–143.
18. Davidoff AM, Hebra A, Kerr J, Stafford PW. Laparoscopic oophorectomy in children. J Laparoendosc Surg 1996; 6 (suppl 1):S115–S119.
19. van der Zee DC, van Seumeren IG, Bax KM, Rovekamp MH, ter Gunne AJ. Laparoscopic approach to surgical management of ovarian cysts in the newborn. J Pediatr Surg 1995; 30:42–43.
20. Dolgin SE. Ovarian masses in the newborn. Semin Pediatr Surg 2000; 9(3):121–127.
21. Germain M, Rarick T, Robins E. Management of intermittent ovarian torsion by laparoscopic oophoropexy. Obstet Gynecol 1996; 88(4):715–717.
22. Wang PH, Lee WL, Chao HT, Yuan CC. Disseminated carcinomatosis after laparoscopic surgery for presumably benign ruptured ovarian teratoma. Eur J Obstet Gynecol Reprod Biol 2000; 89(1):89–91.

8

Renal Cryosurgery

David Y. Chan and Ronald Rodriguez

James Buchanan Brady Urological Institute, Johns Hopkins Medical Institute, Baltimore, Maryland, USA

With the advent of improved abdominal imaging over the last two decades, the proportion of incidentally discovered renal cell carcinoma (RCC) has reached nearly 50–60% (1–4). During the same time, interest in minimally invasive alternatives for surgical ablation of renal neoplasms has also risen. Historically, radical nephrectomy has been the standard for the treatment of RCC (5,6). Recent studies, however, have demonstrated that nephron-sparing nephrectomy or partial nephrectomies are also effective in the management of smaller RCCs (<4 cm) (7–9). However, both are open procedures and require abdominal or flank incisions that can result in significant patient morbidity and a substantial period of convalescence (10).

Several studies have suggested that small renal tumors <3 cm may have a low biologic malignant potential, and select patients with small renal tumors may not need or even desire extirpative surgery (11–14). Though still experimental, cryosurgery may represent a rational alternative for the treatment of these patients.

INTRODUCTION/HISTORY

Cryotherapy refers to the use of freezing temperatures for the treatment of various conditions. Renal cryosurgery is the use of subzero temperatures for *in situ* destruction of kidney tissue. James Arnott first applied iced salt solutions ($\sim -20°C$) to freeze advanced breast and cervical cancer. With this technique, Arnott was able to reduce the size of tumors and ameliorate pain in his patients. However, despite the introduction of solidified carbon dioxide ($-78.5°C$) and liquid oxygen ($-182.9°C$) during the early 1900s, cryosurgery was limited only to topical applications. Without significant improvements in cryogenics and poor hypothermic control, cryosurgery was not considered to be safe or practical (15,16).

During the 1960s, Irving Cooper, a neurosurgeon, introduced a modern automated cryosurgical apparatus that could deliver cryotherapy in a controlled manner. He helped develop a vacuum-insulated liquid nitrogen cooled probe ($-196°C$) for neurosurgical applications. The Joule–Thomson effect describes the rapid cooling that results from the rapid phase change of highly compressed liquid nitrogen expanding through a restricted orifice to a gaseous state (17). This development allowed modern cryosurgery to be effective and practical. Early applications have included cryothalamectomy for the treatment of Parkinson's disease and other neuromuscular disorders (18,19). With these advances, resurgence in cryosurgery began for the treatment of benign conditions including Ménière's disease, hemangiomas, hemorrhoids, and retinal detachment. The use of cryotherapy in other clinical conditions such as visceral cancer has also evolved. However, limitations in accurate tumor imaging and ice ball control restricted the effective application of cryosurgery for deeper structures.

Although the biology of cryosurgery has been known for decades, only recently have advances in technology and imaging permitted its clinical utility (17,20). Intraoperative ultrasound and improved control in the volume, temperature, and thawing of tissue have been the major advances during this past decade.

As a result, cryosurgery has proven to be efficacious in the treatment of colorectal hepatic metastases (21,22). However, applications of cryosurgery in prostatic (23–27) and renal malignancies are still under evaluation (28–35).

PRINCIPLES OF CRYOSURGERY

Pathophysiology of Cryosurgery

Active freezing and passive thawing describe the two phases of tissue destruction during cryosurgery. The freezing phase is performed rapidly with the generation of an ice ball with a core temperature of $-196°C$. Passive thawing is performed more slowly for maximum effect (36). Cellular destruction from the freeze process results from complex direct and indirect physiologic mechanisms. Aside from the direct physical disruption of the cellular membranes, proteins, and intracellular organelles from ice crystals, there are also indirect effects of microvascular thrombosis, osmotic dehydration, and cellular anoxia during the freeze process, which may also extend beyond the physical ice ball (37–39). The histological sequela acutely is coagulative necrosis. With time, chronic fibrosis, scarring, and collagen deposition replace the damaged tissue.

Contact vs. Puncture Cryoablation

Most large-animal studies use the puncture technique for cryoablation (40). Since the freeze process is dependent on the total surface area of contact, contact cryoablation requires more time to ablate the same volume of tissue as puncture cryoablation. Although less bleeding occurs with contact cryoablations, the cryolesions generated are more peripheral and less able to penetrate into deeper tissues (41,42). In one study, the size of the puncture lesions was nearly twice that of the contact lesion (41). Furthermore, the puncture technique permits simpler monitoring and maintaining of the probe position than contact cryoablation. All human clinical cryoablation series have used the puncture technique. Puncture cryoablation should be the preferred method of ablation. Histologically, however, there are no differences in the cryolesions generated by contact or puncture cryoablation (41).

Probe Size and Required Temperature for Successful Cryoablation

Early studies in mouse tumor models already demonstrated significant cure rate differences at a lower cryoprobe tip temperature of $-180°C$ (43). Furthermore, not only did a larger tip-to-tumor contact area accelerate the freezing rate, but it was also found to improve tumor control as compared with probes with a smaller surface area (43). The 3 and 4.8 mm cryoprobes are the more common cryoprobes used at present for renal cryosurgery. Smaller 2–3 mm cryoprobes have recently been introduced for both open and percutaneous renal cryoablation

(34). Preliminary results demonstrate similar efficacy as compared to larger probes. However, multiple punctures are required to ablate similar size lesions.

Ultrasound and direct visualization can estimate the location of the edge of the ice ball. Unfortunately, this information does not provide any physical measurement of tissue temperature. Furthermore, ultrasonography does not provide any images beyond the near edge of the ice ball, as a complete posterior acoustic shadowing will blind any structures beyond the near ice surface (17). Thermocouples have been used to correlate tissue temperature and the ultrasound image. The hyperechoic rim of the advancing edge of freezing tissue seen in the ultrasonic image has been estimated to be 0°C (17). The temperature 3–4 mm inside the edge of the ice ball has been estimated to be −20°C (44).

One controversy surrounding cryoablation is what final temperature is necessary for tissue ablation. From *in vitro* studies, the −40°C isotherm is believed to be the critical temperature for effective cryotherapy (43). Uchida et al. used an *in vitro* renal cancer cell line (NC-65) to examine cell viability after 60 min of cooling at various temperatures. In renal cancer cells cooled down to −10°C, 95% of the cell line was still viable. Only when the temperature reached −20°C to −30°C was there a dramatic decrease in cell viability. Only 15% of cancer cells were viable at −20°C. Cooling test data from this study suggested that tissue temperature should be below −20°C to achieve necrosis of the renal cancer cell. The −40°C isotherm should be the target temperature at the edge of the lesion.

Depending on the probe size, the −40°C isotherm is usually 60% of the distance from the probe to the edge of the ice ball, that is, ~8–10 mm from the ice boundary of a 3 cm ice ball. The location of the −40°C isotherm, however, will vary depending on the rate of cooling of the tissue. A rapid cooling rate will move the isotherm toward the periphery or the ice edge (17). If a rapid freeze is implemented, highly efficient probes cooled to −196°C can move the −40°C isotherm to 5–6 mm inside the border of a 6 cm ice ball lesion. If a rapid freeze technique is used and the visible edge of the ice ball exceeds the tumor by 1 cm, then all margins of the tumors should be below the −40°C isotherm.

Heat Sink Phenomenon and the Need for Renal Artery Occlusion

The process of cryoablation is not tissue specific. Various tissues may have different sensitivities to the freeze process. The extraction of heat or the cooling of the targeted tissue is dependent on the temperature of the cryoprobe, the area of contact of the freezing surface, and the tissue thermal conductivity (43). Differences between tissue resistances to cooling are also dependent on the distance from large blood vessels. This phenomenon is also known as the heat sink effect. A constant supply of warm blood circulating nearby and diffusing thermal energy to the lesion can inhibit the freeze process. Theoretically, this heat sink or thermal conduction can affect the rate of cooling and the size of the cryoablation and prolong the time needed to reach any given temperature.

Uchida et al. (45) studied the effect of warm perfusion on cryoablation. Two human kidneys with RCC were examined *ex vivo* after radical nephrectomy. Both tumors were hypervascular and ~5.0 cm in diameter. The kidneys were submerged into 40°C water tanks, and a cryoprobe was placed into the center of each tumor. Thermocouples were also placed 1 and 2 cm away from the cryoprobe to measure the effective temperature. To examine the role of thermal conduction on cooling, one kidney was perfused with saline at 40°C via the renal artery at 400 cc/min while the other kidney was not. The temperature in the tumor without irrigation reached −45°C in the areas 2 cm away from the probe after 15 min. The temperature in the tumor with irrigation fell more slowly and reached −8°C at the same area after 30 min. Uchida et al. (45) suggested that perhaps embolization of the renal artery may be necessary prior to treating hypervascular tumors. Nakada et al. (41) examined the role of selective embolization with puncture cryotherapy in a porcine model and suggested that selective embolization may be useful in the treatment of larger, central lesions.

These reports conflict with other studies. Campbell et al. (46) did not find any practical advantage in renal artery occlusion prior to cryosurgery. In a solitary kidney canine model, cryoablations were performed with or without concomitant renal artery occlusion. Renal artery occlusion decreased the time required to reach the target temperature, but it did not alter the freeze process. Some *in vivo* experimental evidence from hepatic cryoablation has also demonstrated that complete perivascular and intralesional necrosis near large vessels is possible without vascular occlusion or embolization (47).

Cryoablations of renal hilar lesions have not been specifically addressed. Since all segmental renal arteries are end arteries with no collateral circulation, cryoablation with embolization near the renal hilum, such as the central intraparenchymal lesion, can be precarious. Some animal studies with cryoablation alone have demonstrated a wedge-shaped infarction pattern, suggesting that thromboses of major vascular segmental vessels can occur (48). Cryosurgery with embolization near the renal hilum could potentially thrombose a significant portion of the kidney and would not be considered as nephron sparing. Cryoablation of central lesions should be avoided. Currently, for peripheral lesions, occlusion or embolization of the renal artery provides no practical advantage.

Feasibility of Cryosurgery

Although the histological and ultrastructural effects of cryosurgery in the rat kidney were already described in 1981, the feasibility of focal renal ablation with cryosurgery and the ability of a solitary kidney to tolerate cryoinjury was first demonstrated by Barone in 1988 (48,49). Renal cryoablations were performed in a solitary kidney rabbit model (48). The cryolesions were followed for up to 8 weeks. Although maximal renal dysfunction occurred at 3 days, all renal function returned to normal gradually. This was also accompanied by compensatory renal hypertrophy of the surrounding uninjured parenchyma. Initially, the cryolesions affected 40% of the kidney after 24 h. By 8 weeks, the lesions evolved to a fibrotic lesion, involving only 20% of the kidney (48). This study demonstrated that a solitary kidney could tolerate profound cryoinjury and recover normal function by compensatory renal hypertrophy.

Other animal models including rats (49), rabbits (48,50), dogs (46,42,51), sheep (52), and pigs (29,41,53,54) have been used by various investigators to study cryosurgery. All studies have consistently demonstrated the ability of renal cryosurgery to destroy normal renal parenchyma. In general, the frozen kidney becomes necrotic after 7 days and progresses to scar contraction after 12 weeks. The effect of cryosurgery is essentially an autonephrectomy. The time to complete resorption varies between series.

Intraoperative Monitoring of Cryoablation

The intraoperative monitoring of cryoablation with a computed tomography (CT) scan was described during the early 1980s (55). However, given the limitation of the imaging modality and the absence of thermal information, intraoperative CT imaging has not been used to guide cryosurgery. Onik et al. (51) recommended the use of ultrasound as a potential modality to monitor cryolesions intraoperatively. In their study, freezing results in a hyperechoic rim with posterior acoustic shadowing. As the freeze progresses, this rim increases in size. Although ultrasonography does not offer temperature data, good correlation between gross visible ice ball size and hyperechoic rim was found. Intraoperative ultrasound can guide the cryoprobe to the target deep tissue and monitor the accuracy and extent of freezing accurately.

Although intraoperative ultrasound can visualize renal cryosurgery and identify the borders of the frozen region as a hyperechoic rim created by the interface between frozen and unfrozen tissue, the $-40°C$ isotherm must still be estimated. Consequently, the observable visual edge of the ice ball does not predict cell death (54). Only temperature monitoring using thermocouples could consistently demonstrate cell death.

Ultrasound of the thawed cryolesion also appears hyperechoic as compared with the unfrozen kidney. This has important implications for intraoperative monitoring during the second freeze process, as the hyperechoic thaw cryolesion may mask the location of the true edge of the second freeze hyperechoic rim. Overall, Onik et al. (51) found good correlation between the ultrasound and autopsy measurements of the cryolesions obtained. Intraoperative ultrasonography plays an integral role in monitoring renal cryosurgery today.

More recently, the feasibility of percutaneous cryoablation monitoring using magnetic resonance imaging (MRI) has been examined by Shingleton and colleagues (34,56). In both animal and human studies, MRI provides successful probe placement and accurate monitoring of ice ball formation. Since MRI allows for multiplanar imaging, it may be also helpful for cryoablation of intraparenchymatous tumors. If MR thermometry can be coupled with image guidance, percutaneous cryosurgery may supplant open and laparoscopic procedures.

Number of Freeze Cycles

Several studies in the urologic literature have questioned the value of double freezing in their normal renal parenchyma animal model cryoablation studies (29,47,52). Repeat cycles of freeze–thaw have consistently demonstrated superior cure rates in other studies using animal tumor models (57). The current data support the use of more than one freeze–thaw cycle to ensure maximum lethality of cryotherapy (39,57–59). In addition, double freezing has become the rule in the treatment of hepatic malignancies with good success (60).

Historically, the application of cryoablation for treatment of hepatic metastasis has used a double-freeze technique (60). Several studies have found no histological differences between the single- and double-freeze technique (29,41,47,52). Bishoff et al. (29) noted that the double-freeze technique resulted in larger ablated lesions. The limitations of all data using the single-freeze technique involve the use of normal tissues for cryoablation. Extrapolation of data from ablation of normal parenchyma in animal models to human cancers is problematic. Data supporting the use of the double-freeze technique derive from *in vitro* tissue cultures of hepatic and renal tumor cell lines (45). Similarly, *in vitro* models are also inadequate, as some have argued that to obtain reproducible necrosis, *in vivo* tissue may not require exposure to temperatures as low as are needed for *in vitro* cell studies (61). Unfortunately, there are no adequate large-animal renal tumor models.

VX-2, a cervical papilloma, has been used to mimic renal tumors in rabbits. The tumor is extremely aggressive and by definition, when implanted into the kidney, metastatic. To date, only one study has used VX-2 tumor to model the efficacy of cryosurgery for renal tumor ablation (50). Nakada et al. randomized 24 rabbits with renal implants of VX-2 into three groups: observation, nephrectomy, and *single*-freeze cryoablation. In this study, all animals in the observation group developed lung and liver metastases with aggressive local invasion. There was no significant difference in survival or development of metastasis between the nephrectomy and cryoablation groups. Although VX-2 is a poor renal tumor model, the results with single-freeze cryoablation suggest a potential role and efficacy of cryosurgery as a potential minimally invasive nephron-sparing modality. Until more definite data become available, however, double cycles of rapid freeze with slow thaw should be the standard for renal cryosurgery.

Surgical Margins and Pathologic Diagnosis

One major drawback to cryoablation is the absence of tissue diagnosis. Although intraoperative biopsy can be obtained at the time of the procedure, renal biopsies for renal masses are often inadequate and are prone to false negatives and false positives. Dechet et al. (62) confirmed these findings even with open biopsy. Although there was a high positive predictive value for carcinoma, benign lesions are often misdiagnosed. This has tremendous implications for patient follow-up and evaluation of the efficacy of cryosurgery. Furthermore, there is no method for ensuring that *all* margins of tumors are ablated and are negative for viable tumor. Subsequently, it is paramount that all cryoablations must ablate beyond the edge of the tumor.

One other concern includes the involvement of the collecting system. Although Gill and colleagues (63) have recently demonstrated in a porcine model that direct injury to the collecting system did not result in urinary leak or fistula, involvement of the collecting system and renal hemorrhage have been noted in other animal studies and are potential concerns (41,46,53).

CLINICAL STUDIES

Uchida et al. (45) reported the first percutaneous approach for renal cryoablation in two patients with advanced RCC. Under general anesthesia and ultrasound guidance, percutaneous puncture was performed in the center of the renal tumor. The cryoprobe was placed into the tract after it was dilated to 24F and a Teflon sheath was placed to prevent heat conduction. Using thermocouples for real-time monitoring, the tumor was cooled to $-20°C$. A nephrostomy tube was inserted after the procedure. Although both patients expired, at 5 and at 10 months after the procedure, improvements in Karnofsky performance scale and reduction in tumor size were noted in both patients.

Delworth et al. (64) also presented the use of cryotherapy in two patients with tumors in their solitary kidneys. One patient had multifocal RCC, while the second patient had angiomyolipoma. Both patients underwent open cryosurgery with double-freeze technique. Both patients had stable creatinine postoperatively and tolerated the procedure without complications. With 1 month of follow-up, Delworth found that cryoablation was feasible with minimal loss of renal function.

The largest published human renal cryosurgery experience to date is from a Cleveland Clinic (28,31). They have performed over 34 renal cryoablations in 32 patients without complications. All lesions were small (<4 cm) peripheral, exophytic, and solid. The indications for cryosurgery included solitary kidney, renal dysfunction, suspected renal metastasis, and compromised contralateral renal unit. Tumor size less than 4 cm accounted for a significant number of patients as the only indication for cryosurgery.

Postoperative renal function at 24 h was unchanged in their study. There was no evidence of urine leakage. One patient was noted to have a perirenal hematoma that was managed conservatively. With a mean follow-up of 8.5 months, there has been no evidence of local tumor growth or port site recurrences. Using MRI, concentric nonenhancing defects in cryoablated areas were seen. After 3 months, there was a 40% reduction in the size of the cryolesions.

These were consistent with postcryoablation scars. Biopsies of these cryolesion scars at 3 months in 12 patients have been negative for malignancy.

McGinnis and Strup (30) also recently reported their experience with renal cryosurgery. Between September 1997 and July 1999, 10 patients underwent laparoscopic retroperitoneal cryoablation of renal tumors. In their series, patients who were candidates for partial nephrectomy were also candidates for cryosurgery. Intraoperative ultrasound was used to access renal tumor and cryoablation. Renal biopsies were obtained. Five of 10 were diagnosed as RCC. Two biopsies were indeterminate. The remaining three biopsies revealed angiomyolipoma, oncocytoma, and focal pyelonephritis. No complications or delayed bleeding were noted postoperatively. With a mean follow-up of 11 months, all lesions had diminished in size. There was also presence of residual scar tissue on follow-up CT scans in their series.

Rukstalis et al. (35) also reported their series of open renal cryoablations in 29 patients. The median lesion size was 2.2 cm. Five patients (17%) developed serious adverse events. Of the patients with a median follow-up of 16 months, 91.3% demonstrated a complete radiographic response with only a residual scar or small, nonenhancing cyst. One biopsy-proven local recurrence was found in their study.

Rodiguez et al. (32) reported eight patients who had been treated with renal cryosurgery. All tumors were small (<3 cm) and exophytic. All patients were offered traditional treatments, but they did not want radical nephrectomy or partial nephrectomy. The mean age of the patients was 64 years. Renal biopsies revealed six RCCs. Two biopsies were indeterminate. The mean tumor size was 2.2 cm. The mean freeze time was 15 min. With a mean follow-up of 14 months, there were no changes in serum creatinine. All follow-up CT scans revealed significant reduction of tumors. Two patients had self-limiting postoperative complications, of which only one was symptomatic. The symptomatic patient had a transient exacerbation of motor weakness from a prior cerebrovascular accident (CVA). Her symptoms resolved spontaneously with appropriate supportive care. One asymptomatic patient was found to have a pelvic vein thrombosis on follow-up CT scan. Recently, one of the patients was found to have growth of the postcryoablation scar after 1 year. Despite the radiological evidence of recurrence, that patient has deferred any surgical intervention. The reason for these failures is unclear, but they could have resulted from inadequate tumor freezing or poor tumor targeting.

Shingleton et al. presented their data on percutaneous cryoablation with MR guidance. Twenty patients with 22 renal tumors were treated. The mean tumor size was 3.0 cm. With a mean follow-up of 9.1 months, no radiographic evidence of disease recurrence or new tumor development was found. However, one patient had evidence of persistent tumor that required re-treatment. The only complication noted was a superficial wound abscess.

Levin et al. (65) reported one recurrence in 22 patients with postlaparoscopic renal cryoablation biopsy. According to the abstract, the patient had a negative biopsy at 6 months, but was rebiopsied at 9 months for a suspicious nodule on a subsequent MRI scan. RCC was demonstrated at that biopsy. The patient underwent radical nephrectomy and was found to have a 1.3 cm focus of clear cell renal carcinoma.

Application of renal cryoablation in clinical studies appears to be a safe technique for the destruction of solid renal masses. However, inadequate freezing is the major concern and may result in local disease persistence requiring further intervention. In the review of the literature, four recurrences have occurred. Frequent radiographic follow-up is paramount as the slow growth rate of small renal cancers necessitates prolonged radiologic follow-up. Further clinical evaluation is essential before renal cryoablation can be considered an acceptable alternative for the treatment of renal cancer.

PATIENT SELECTION, INDICATIONS, AND SUITABILITY OF CRYOSURGERY

Careful patient selection is paramount, as renal cryosurgery is still an experimental procedure. All patients should be counseled about the alternative nature of cryoablation and should be first offered traditional methods for the management of renal tumors, that is, open or laparoscopic radical nephrectomy, and partial nephrectomy, and even the possibility of observation alone. Since most lesions do not resolve completely and leave a postcryoablation scar, patients should also be advised about the need for frequent follow-up to ensure no interval tumor growth. And given the novel technique, if the cryoablation procedure fails to control the renal tumor, the patient may need further surgical intervention.

Given the complexity and the novelty of cryoablation, this procedure should be limited to older patients with small, exophytic tumors (<3 cm) who desire intervention but not radical or partial nephrectomy. Younger, healthy patients should be informed potentially against cryosurgery in lieu of traditional extirpative procedures since they will have a longer life expectancy and be subjected to a lifetime of radiologic follow-up. An ideal candidate would be an elderly patient with multiple medical problems and a solitary kidney and a small peripheral tumor <3 cm who does not want radical or partial nephrectomy. However, as with any novel procedure, the indications are still evolving.

OPERATIVE TECHNIQUE

To maintain the minimally invasive modality of cryosurgery, the laparoscopic technique should be used. The approach should be dictated by the location of the tumor and the surgeon's comfort. If an open procedure is utilized, it is approached similar to open transperitoneal or extraperitoneal partial nephrectomy (35). The renal unit is exposed. Intraoperative ultrasound is used to rule out other lesions. Once the specific renal mass has been identified, the portion of Gerota's fasica overlying the tumor is excised and sent for histologic analysis.

A biopsy is obtained for tissue diagnosis. A variable number of cryoprobes are placed under ultrasound guidance so that the area of cryoablation exceeds the tumor by 1 cm. Double rapid freeze and slow thaw is prefered. Larger lesions will require multiple ablations to encompass the entire lesion. Once the freeze process is complete, the cryoprobes are removed and the entry sites are occluded with thrombin soaked Gelfoam.

If the laparoscopic approach is utilized, the transperitoneal approach provides the greatest amount of working space. In our experience, we reserve the retroperitoneal approach for upper pole and posterior medial tumors. The retroperitoneal approach is also safe and feasible and has been favored by others (28,30).

After general endotracheal anesthesia is obtained, the patient is placed in the modified ipsilateral flank position. A warming blanket is placed. The patient is given antibiotics before the procedure begins. For a small, left lower pole exophytic renal tumor, we would use the three-port technique (Fig. 8.1). A Veress needle is used to obtain intraperitoneal access. The abdomen is insufflated with CO_2 to a pressure of 15–20 mmHg. The laparoscope is inserted at the level of the iliac crest, lateral to the rectus muscle, using the Visiport device (US Surgical, Stamford, CT). The two additional trocars, one at the umbilicus and one at two finger breadths subxyphoid, are placed under direct vision.

The first incision is made at the line of Toldt (Fig. 8.2). The peritoneum and bowel are reflected medially to expose the kidney. Care is taken not to enter Gerota's fasica. Once the kidney has been isolated, as in the open procedure, a laparoscopic ultrasound is used to scan the kidney and identify the exact location of the tumor and rule out the presence of undetected masses. Once the location of the tumor has been identified (Fig. 8.3), the fat anterior to the tumor is incised sharply and sent as an intact specimen to rule out tumor invasion (T3a). Next,

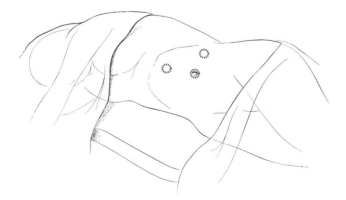

Figure 8.1 Patient is placed in a modified flank position. For a laparoscopic transperitoneal left renal cryosurgery, the patient is in a 45° oblique position utilizing three ports.

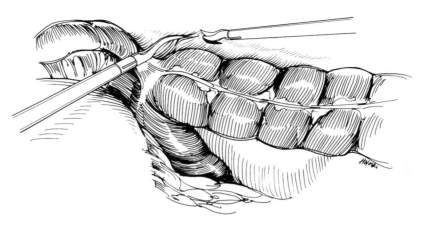

Figure 8.2 The line of Toldt is sharply incised. The descending colon is reflected medially to expose the kidney.

the renal tumor is biopsied. The specimen is sent for pathological diagnosis. Using the same biopsy tract, the cryoprobe is placed in the tumor under ultrasound guidance to ensure that the probe is placed properly in the tumor.

The area is inspected again prior to initiation of the cryoprocess to ensure that no tissue can be frozen nearby (Fig. 8.4). The initial freeze is started slowly. This allows for better control of the initial "stick". If the initial freeze is started at the maximum power, no adjustment can be made, and any torque can result in excessive bleeding during the thaw phase. When the probe is "stuck" and in the proper position, the freeze process can be maximized to allow for a rapid freeze. Ultrasound can be used to visualize the intraparenchymal edge of the ice ball. Care must be taken to avoid contact with other structures during the freeze–thaw process. This usually takes 10–15 min depending on the size of the lesion.

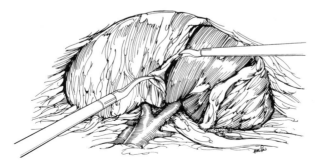

Figure 8.3 Only the perinephric tissue is dissected from the kidney. The perinephric tissue over the lower pole tumor is removed separately and sent to pathology to rule out perinephric extension.

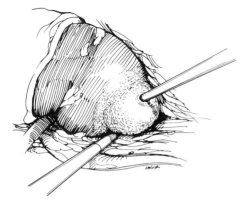

Figure 8.4 After renal biopsy of the tumor is performed, the cryosurgical probe is inserted into the biopsy tract. The ice ball is extended approximately 1 cm beyond the tumor edge.

When the edge of the ice ball has extended 1 cm beyond the tumor the freeze process can be stopped. Thawing is allowed passively. The slow thaw is an important factor in obtaining cell death. Once the freeze–thaw cycle is complete, a second freeze–thaw cycle is repeated to ensure adequate tissue destruction. Once the second cycle is completed, the probe is removed carefully. A Gelfoam plug is inserted into the biopsy/probe site to tamponade bleeding (Fig. 8.5). Argon beam may also be helpful in obtaining hemostasis if there is any capsular bleeding. Once hemostasis is obtained, the Gerota's fasica is reapproximated and the kidney is retroperitonealized. Significant adhesions can develop if the kidney is not retroperitonealized (29). After the procedure is completed, the abdominal insufflation is released. All trocar ports are removed under direct vision and are closed using the Carter–Thomason device. The skin trocar sites are reapproximated with absorbable subcutaneous suture.

Postoperatively, patients are slowly advanced to a regular diet, usually by the second or third postoperative day. Since cryosurgery is still experimental we recommend obtaining an abdominal CT scan on postoperative day 1. This ensures that the tumor is ablated completely and provides a baseline for future follow-up. We recommend frequent interval imaging during the first year, at 3, 6, and 12 months. CT scans should be performed annually thereafter. If there is any evidence of tumor growth or incomplete tumor ablation, surgical extirpation of the tumor should be recommended to the patient.

RISKS AND BENEFITS

If renal cryoablation proves to be efficacious, the benefits of this novel minimally invasive modality are tremendous. It is a minimally invasive nephron-sparing

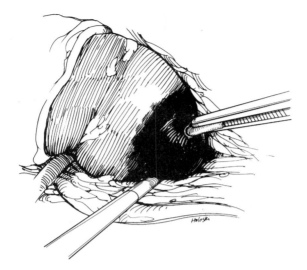

Figure 8.5   After a double freeze–thaw is completed, a Gelfoam plug is inserted into the biopsy/probe site to tamponade bleeding.

alternative to standard surgery. To date, the patient morbidity of the procedure, though not negligible, has been minimal. Morbidity may also be further reduced with a percutaneous approach (53). If percutaneous cryosurgery for small renal tumors proves to be successful, it will mark a new era in surgical advances.

Until that time however, cryosurgery is still experimental and has not yet been proven. Since only tumor biopsies are obtained, definitive pathological diagnoses are not possible. It is also not possible to evaluate surgical margins. Given that several recurrences have been discovered and that cryolesions resorb slowly to residual scars, patients are committed to frequent radiological follow-ups.

CONCLUSIONS

Limited clinical trials in selected patients have allowed cautious optimism for renal cryoablation. Longer follow-up, however, is essential to determine the ultimate efficacy of renal cryosurgery. Cryosurgery of the kidney is still experimental. Although early data from human trials are promising, until proven, traditional surgery should be performed when possible.

REFERENCES

1. Jayson M, Sanders H. Increased incidence of serendipitously discovered renal cell carcinoma. Urology 1998; 51:203–205.

2. Bretheau D, Koutani A, Lechevallier E, Coulange C. A French national epidemiologic survey on renal cell carcinoma: Oncology Committee of the Association Francaise d'Urologie. Cancer 1998; 82:538–544.

3. Gudbjartsson T, Einarsson GV, Magnusson J. A population-based analysis of survival and incidental diagnosing of renal cell carcinoma in Iceland, 1971–1990. Scand J Urol Nephrol 1996; 30:451–455.

4. Sweeny JP, Thornhill JA, Graiger R, McDermott TE, Butler MR. Incidentally detected renal cell carcinoma: pathological features, survival trends, and implications for treatment. Br J Urol 1996; 78:351–353.

5. Robson CJ, Churchill BM, Anderson W. The results of radical nephrectomy for renal cell carcinoma. J Urol 1969; 101(3):297–301.

6. Skinner DG, Colvin RB, Vermillion CD, Pfister RC, Leadbetter WF. Diagnosis and management of renal cell carcinoma. A clinical and pathologic study of 309 cases. Cancer 1971; 28(5):1165–1177.

7. Lerner SE, Hawkins CA, Blute ML, Grabner A, Wollan PC, Eickholt JT, Zincke H. Disease outcome in patients with low stage renal cell carcinoma treated with nephron sparing or radical surgery. J Urol 1996; 155(6):1868–1873.

8. Licht MR, Novick AC. Nephron sparing surgery for renal cell carcinoma. J Urol 1993; 149(1):1–7.

9. Butler BP, Novick AC, Miller DP, Campbell SA, Licht MR. Management of small unilateral renal cell carcinomas: radical versus nephron-sparing surgery. Urology 1995; 45(1):34–40.

10. Campbell SC, Novick AC. Surgical technique and morbidity of elective partial nephrectomy. Semin Urol Oncol 1995; 13(4):281–287.

11. Johnsen JA, Hellsten S. Lymphatogenous spread of renal cell carcinoma: an autopsy study. J Urol 1997; 157(2):450–453.

12. Levine E, Huntrakoon M, Wetzel LH. Small renal neoplasms: clinical, pathologic, and imaging features. Am J Roentgenol 1989; 153(1):69–73.

13. Bosniak MA. Observation of small incidentally detected renal masses. Semin Urol Oncol 1995; 13(4):267–272.

14. Bosniak MA, Birnbaum BA, Krinsky GA, Waisman J. Small renal parenchymal neoplasms: further observations on growth. Radiology 1995; 197(3):589–597.

15. Pusey WA. The use of carbon dioxide snow in the treatment of nevi and other lesions of the skin. J Am Med Assoc 1907; 49:371–377.

16. Irvine HG, Turnacliff DD. Liquid oxygen in dermatology. Arch Dermatol Syphild 1929; 19:270–280.

17. Baust J, Gage AA, Ma H, Zhang CM. Minimally invasive cryosurgery—technological advances. Cryobiology 1997; 34(4):373–384.

18. Cooper IS. Cryogenic surgery: a new method of destruction or extirpation of benin or malignant tissues. N Engl J Med 1963; 268:743–749.

19. Cooper IS. Relief of intention tremor of multiple sclerosis by thalamic surgery. J Am Med Assoc 1967; 199(10):689–694.

20. Lutzeyer W, Lymberopoulos S, Breining H, et al. Experimental cryosurgery of the kidney. Langenbecks Arch Chir 1968; 322:843–847.

21. Korpan NN. Hepatic cryosurgery for liver metastases. Long-term follow-up. Ann Surg 1997; 225:193–201.

22. McCarty TM, Kuhn JA. Cryotherapy for liver tumors. Oncology (Huntingt) 1998; 12(7):979–987.

23. Connolly JA, Shinohara K, Carroll PR. Cryosurgery for locally advanced (T3) pros-
    tate cancer. Semin Urol Oncol 1997; 15:244–249.
24. Koppie TM, Shinohara K, Grossfeld GD, Presti JC Jr, Carroll PR. The efficacy of
    cryosurgical ablation of prostate cancer: the University of California, San Francisco
    experience. J Urol 1999; 162(2):427–432.
25. Gould RS. Total cryosurgery of the prostate versus standard cryosurgery versus
    radical prostatectomy: comparison of early results and the role of transurethral resec-
    tion in cryosurgery. J Urol 1999; 162(5):1653–1657.
26. Chin JL, Pautler SE, Mouraviev V, Touma N, Moore K, Downey DB. Results of
    salvage cryoablation of the prostate after radiation: identifying predictors of treatment
    failure and complications. J Urol 2001; 165(6):1937–1941.
27. Long JP, Bahn D, Lee F, Shinohara K, Chinn DO, Macaluso JN Jr. Five-year
    retrospective, multi-institutional pooled analysis of cancer-related outcomes after
    cryosurgical ablation of the prostate. Urology 2001; 57(3):518–523.
28. Gill IS, Novick AC, Soble JJ, Sung GT, Remer EM, Hale J, O'Malley CM. Laparo-
    scopic renal cryoablation: initial clinical series. Urology 1998; 52(4):543–551.
29. Bishoff JT, Chen RB, Lee BR, Chan DY, Huso D, Rodriguez R, Kavoussi LR,
    Marshall FF. Laparoscopic renal cryoablation: acute and long-term clinical, radio-
    graphic, and pathologic effects in an animal model and application in a clinical
    trial. J Endourol 1999; 13(4):233–239.
30. McGinnis DE, Strup SE. Retroperitoneal laparoscopic cryoablation of renal tumors:
    preliminary results. P100. 57th Annual Meeting of the Mid-Atlantic Section of
    American Urological Association, Hilton Head, SC, 2000.
31. Gill IS, Novick AC, Meraney AM, Chen RN, Hobart MG, Sung GT, Hale J,
    Schweizer DK, Remer EM. Laparoscopic renal cryoablation in 32 patients. Urology
    2000; 56(5):748–753.
32. Rodriguez R, Chan DY, Bishoff JT, Chen RC, Kavoussi LR, Marshall FF. Renal abla-
    tive cryosurgery in select patients with peripheral renal masses. Urology 2000;
    55(1):25–30.
33. Johnson DB, Nakada SY. Laparoscopic cryoablation for renal-cell cancer. J Endourol
    2000; 14(10):873–878; discussion 878–879.
34. Shingleton WB, Sewell PE Jr. Percutaneous renal tumor cryoablation with magnetic
    resonance imaging guidance. J Urol 2001; 165(3):773–776.
35. Rukstalis DB, Khorsandi M, Garcia FU, Hoenig DM, Cohen JK. Clinical experience
    with open renal cryoablation. Urology 2001; 57(1):34–39.
36. Gage AA, Baust J. Mechanisms of tissue injury in cryosurgery. Cryobiology 1998;
    37(3):171–186.
37. Carpenter RJ III, Snyder GG III. Cryosurgery: theory and application to head and neck
    neoplasia. Head Neck Surg 1979; 2:129–141.
38. Rubinsky B, Lee CY, Bastacky J, Onik G. The process of freezing and the mechanism
    of damage during hepatic cryosurgery. Cryobiology 1990; 27(1):85–97.
39. Gill W, Frazier J, Carter DC. Repeated freeze-thaw cycles in cryosurgery. Nature
    1968; 219:410–413.
40. Nakada SY. Newer techniques for surgical ablation of renal neoplasms. Contemp
    Urol 1999; 11(10):68–80.
41. Nakada SY, Lee FT Jr, Warner TF, Chosy SG, Moon TD. Laparoscopic renal
    cryotherapy in swine: comparison of puncture cryotherapy preceded by arterial embo-
    lization and contact cryotherapy. J Endourol 1998; 12(6):567–573.

42. Stephenson RA, King DK, Rohr LR. Renal cryoablation in a canine model. Urology 1996; 47(5):772–776.
43. Neel HB III, Ketcham AS, Hammond WG. Requisites for successful cryogenic surgery of cancer. Arch Surg 1971; 102(1):45–48.
44. Saliken J, Cohen J, Miller R, Rothert M. Laboratory evaluation of ice formation around a 3 mm Accuprobe. Cryobiology 1995; 32:285–295.
45. Uchida M, Imaide Y, Sugimoto K, Uehara H, Watanabe H. Percutaneous cryosurgery for renal tumours. Br J Urol 1995; 75(2):132–136.
46. Campbell SC, Krishnamurthi V, Chow G, Hale J, Myles J, Novick AC. Renal cryosurgery: experimental evaluation of treatment parameters. Urology 1998; 52(1):29–33.
47. Weber SM, Lee FT Jr, Chinn DO, Warner T, Chosy SG, Mahvi DM. Perivascular and intralesional tissue necrosis after hepatic cryoablation: results in a porcine model. Surgery 1997; 122(4):742–747.
48. Barone GW, Rodgers BM. Morphologic and functional effects of renal cryoinjury. Cryobiology 1988; 25(4):363–371.
49. Sindelar WF, Javadpour N, Bagley DH. Histological and ultrastructural changes in rat kidney after cryosurgery. J Surg Oncol 1981; 18(4):363–379.
50. Nakada SY, Jerde TJ, Lee FT, Warner T. Efficacy of cryotherapy and nephrectomy in treating implanted VX-2 carcinoma in rabbit kidneys. J Endourol 1999; 13:A13.
51. Onik GM, Reyes G, Cohen JK, Porterfield B. Ultrasound characteristics of renal cryo-surgery. Urology 1993; 42(2):212–215.
52. Cozzi PJ, Lynch WJ, Collins S, Vonthethoff L, Morris DL. Renal cryotherapy in a sheep model; a feasibility study. J Urol 1997; 157:710–712.
53. Long JP, Faller GT. Percutaneous cryoablation of the kidney in a porcine model. Cryobiology 1999; 38(1):89–93.
54. Chosy SG, Nakada SY, Lee FT Jr, Warner TF. Monitoring renal cryosurgery: predictors of tissue necrosis in swine. J Urol 1998; 159(4):1370–1374.
55. Reiser M, Drukier AK, Ultsch B, Feuerbach S. The use of CT in monitoring cryosurgery. S Eur J Radiol 1983; 3(2):123–128.
56. Shingleton WB, Farabaugh P, Hughson M, Sewell PE Jr. Percutaneous cryoablation of porcine kidneys with magnetic resonance imaging monitoring. J Urol 2001; 166(1):289–291.
57. Mascarenhas BA, Ravikumar TS. Experimental basis for hepatic cryotherapy. Semin Surg Oncol 1998; 14(2):110–115.
58. Neel HB III, Ketcham AS, Hammond WG. Cryonecrosis of normal and tumor-bearing rat liver potentiated by inflow occlusion. Cancer 1971; 28:1211–1218.
59. Ravikumar TS, Steele G Jr, Kane R, King V. Experimental and clinical observations on hepatic cryosurgery for colorectal metastasis. Cancer Res 1991; 51(23 Pt 1): 6323–6327.
60. Dilley AV, Dy DY, Warlters A, Copeland S, Gillies AE, Morris RW, Gibb DB, Cook TA, Morris DL. Laboratory and animal model evaluation of the Cryotech LCS 2000 in hepatic cryotherapy. Cryobiology 1993; 30:74–85.
61. Cozzi PJ, Lawson JA, Lynch WJ, Morris DL. Critical temperature for in vivo cryoablation of human prostate cancer in a xenograft model. Br J Urol 1996; 77:89–92.
62. Dechet CB, Sebo T, Farrow G, Blute ML, Engen DE, Zincke H. Prospective analysis of intraoperative frozen needle biopsy of solid renal masses in adults. J Urol 1999; 162(4):1282–1284.

63. Sung GT, Gill IS, Hsu THS, Meraney AM, Reemer E. Effect of intentional cryoinjury to the renal collecting system. J Endourol 1999; 13(S1):A14.
64. Delworth MG, Pisters LL, Fornage BD, von Eschenbach AC. Cryotherapy for renal cell carcinoma and angiomyolipoma. J Urol 1996; 155(1):252–254.
65. Levin HS, Meraney AM, Novick AC, Gill IS. Needle biopsy histology of renal tumors 3–6 months after laparoscopic renal cryoablation. J Urology 2000; 163(4S):53.

9

Cryoablation of the Prostate

Aaron E. Katz and Mohamed A. Ghafar

*Department of Urology, College of Physicians & Surgeons,
Columbia University, New York, New York, USA*

Over the past decade, there has been a strong movement within urologic oncology toward minimally invasive diagnostic procedures as well as therapies. Two prime examples of this for prostate cancer are laparascopic radical prostatectomy and brachytherapy. The goals of minimally invasive therapies for a malignancy of a solid organ are to eradicate the local disease, shorten hospital stay, limit postoperative morbidities, quicken return to daily functions and work, and reduce the overall cost of the procedure. Although some of these therapies are relatively new, they are gaining popularity rather quickly, and several worldwide experiences have demonstrated that they are quite effective in achieving most or all of these goals (1).

Recently, there has been increased interest among urologists in cryosurgical ablation for locally advanced or radiation recurrent prostate cancer (1). Cryosurgery is defined as the *in situ* freezing of a tissue. The goals of cryosurgery for prostate cancer are to ablate the entire gland, rendering the patient free of disease, while preventing the freezing of surrounding structures, such as the bladder, rectum, and external striated sphincter. Currently, the procedure is performed percutaneously, introducing small cryoprobes though the perineal skin into the gland. The placement of the probes is performed using ultrasound guidance. Modern techniques of cryosurgery include an argon-based system to generate lethal ice. This system allows the urologist to monitor the ice ball formation visually by ultrasound and thermally by temperature sensors (2). These devices have dramatically reduced the morbidity of the procedure and have allowed the urologists to determine the endpoints of cryosugery (2). Once the outer freezing edge of the iceball extends beyond the posterior capsule of the gland and into Denonvilleirs' fascia, the freezing process can be stopped, thereby preventing damage to the anterior rectal wall. This has resulted in a significant reduction in rectal fistulas (2). Most current series report a 0–2% incidence of rectal fistulas (2,3)

HISTORY OF CRYOSURGERY

Cryosurgery has been used for the treatment of many benign and malignant conditions. The use of freezing techniques in the treatment of carcinoma began in London during the 1850s when "iced" ($-18°$ to $-22°C$) saline solutions were utilized to treat advanced carcinoma of the breast, uterus, and cervix (4).

In 1907 cryosurgery was utilized in dermatological patients, with the reported cure rate for skin cancer equal to that obtained by surgical excision (5). In recent years, cryosurgery has been utilized for the treatment of a wide variety of diseases, including liver, prostate, and kidney malignancies (5). The first use of transurethral cryosurgical ablation of the prostate in human was reported in 1966 (6). However, several problems became apparent: gross sloughing, severe bladder outlet obstruction, and prolonged hospitalization (6–8). Flocks modified the technique in 1969 to involve the open perineal exposure of the posterior prostate surface with direct application of the cryoprobes (9). This approach produced much less urethral sloughing than the transurethral approach (10). However, effective monitoring of the ice ball in both techniques was inadequate or absent. This caused freezing of the surrounding structures, fistulas, and urinary and fecal incontinence in a significant number of patients undergoing this operation (11,12).

After the development of transrectal ultrasound imaging of the prostate (TRUS), Onik et al. (13) in 1988 described a modification of the technique by placing percutaneous cryoprobes into the prostate under TRUS. The TRUS accurately monitored the propagation of the ice ball and prevented damage of the surrounding structures (14).

MECHANISMS OF TISSUE INJURY IN CRYOSURGERY

To understand the mechanisms of tissue injury in cryosurgery we should under stand the freeze–thaw cycle, which is the critical component of cryosurgery. All cryobiological studies showed that rapid cooling is more destructive. For this reason, in cryosurgery, the cooling rate is always as high as possible in order to produce the lethal intracellular ice.

Mechanisms of Tissue Injury during Freezing Cycles

1. *Direct cell injury*: As temperature falls, the function and structure of cells including their constituents, proteins and lipids, is stressed, cell metabolism progressively fails, and death results. Rapid cooling does not allow time for water to leave the cells, leading to ice crystal formation (15,16), which primarily starts in the extracellular space creating a hyperosmotic extracellular environment, which in turn withdraws water from the cells. The freezing process continues cells shrink, and ice crystal expansion might lead to rupturing of cell membranes (17).

2. *Vascular stasis*: The effect of circulatory stagnation after cold injury is already known from investigations on frostbite. Cellular anoxia is commonly considered to be the main mechanism of injury in cryosurgery. The initial response to the cooling of tissue is vasoconstriction and a decrease in the flow of blood, and finally, the circulation ceases (17).

Mechanisms of Tissue Injury during Thawing Cycles

1. *Recrystallization*: During thawing, ice crystals fuse to form large crystals, which are disruptive to cell membranes. Furthermore as ice melts, the extracellular environment becomes hypotonic and withdraws water from the surrounding tissue, which may also rupture the cell membrane. The damaged tissue is subject to continued metabolic derangements during this time (17).

2. *Vascular stasis*: As the tissue thaws and the tissue temperature climbs over 0°C, the circulation returns, now with vasodilatation. The hyperemic response is brief and increased vascular permeability occurs within a few minutes. Edema develops and progresses over a few hours. Changes in the capillary endothelial cells that progress to defects in the endothelial cell junctions have been observed about 2 h after thawing (17).

HISTOPATHOLOGICAL CHANGES AFTER CRYOSURGERY

1. Histopathologically, cryoablated tissues start to show features of irreversible cell death at 1 h. Electron microscopy reveals chromatin condensation, loss of nuclear membrane, partial fragmentation, and thrombi in capillaries and cytoplasmic vacuolization of membranes (18). Light microscopy reveals signs of acute inflammation, vascular congestion, well-defined areas of interstitial hemorrhage, and early coagulation necrosis
2. Granulation tissue, basal cell hyperplasia, cell swelling, focal haemosiderin deposits, and thickening of small nerves are also noted (19).
3. There is marked fibrosis with hyalinization, squamous metaplasia of regenerating duct epithelia, and basal cell hyperplasia of gland acini. Scattered normal ducts with flattened epithelia are present; patent or virtual lumina are occasionally seen. Coagulative necrosis could also be observed in some biopsy fragments obtained 12 months after cryotherapy (19).

ROLE OF HORMONAL THERAPY

The uses of neoadjuvant hormonal therapy prior to cryosurgery is still controversial.We have routinely used hormonal therapy for 3 months prior to cryosurgery for several reasons:

1. Androgen deprivation will lead to decrease in the prostate gland size, which might increase the efficacy of cryosurgery (20).
2. Large gland volume prevents adequate freezing of the prostate, leading to inadequate cell kill (20).
3. Despite negative metastatic evaluation a significant number of patients may have microscopic disease in their peripheral circulation. Hormonal therapy has the additional advantage of clearing this hematogenous micrometastasis, although up to 40% of distant metastases do not respond to hormonal therapy (21)

CRYOSURGICAL TECHNIQUE

1. *Preparation of the patient*: Patients are given a Fleets enema on the morning of the procedure and Flagyl 500 mg IV at the start of the procedure. Cryosurgical ablation of the prostate can be performed under spinal or general anesthesia. The patient is placed in a standard lithotomy position, and the external genitalia, lower abdominal wall, and perineum are draped and prepped in the usual sterile manner.

2. *Placement of sheaths*: Initially, an 18F Foley catheter is placed in the bladder, and the bladder is distended with 300 cc of sterile water. The Foley is left indwelling, clamped to allow the bladder to remain distended, so that the urethra can be visualized under ultrasound. The scrotal skin is then tacked up to the anterior abdominal wall with two small towel clips, allowing the surgeon to have exposure to the perineum. At this point, a transrectal ultrasound is introduced into the rectum, and connected to a brachy-stand. This allows accurate measurements of the gland to be performed using both the transverse and the longitudinal planes. At our institution we have used a B&K 7.5 mHz probe and a Barzell–Whitmore stand.

Recent advances in cryosurgery have led to the generation of a computer-guided cryosurgical system. This system allows the surgeon to input transverse ultrasound images of the gland from the base to the apex in a stepwise manner (22). Once the images are captured, the surgeon can outline the capsule of the gland, urethra, and anterior rectal wall. The computer-guided system will automatically determine the number and placement of cryoprobes required. Typically, a 30–40 g prostate will require six cryoprobes (two anteriorly, two posteriomedially, and two posteriolaterally) (Fig. 9.1). Placement of the individual cryoprobes is performed percutaneously with the aid of a needle and dilator system, known as the FastTrac. This allows the sheaths to be inserted into the gland.

3. *Procedural cystoscopy*: Once all cryosheaths are inserted, the indwelling urethral Foley is removed and a flexible cystoscopy is performed. The flexible scope is passed into the prostatic urethra where inspection of this area is carefully performed. If one or more of the cryosheaths are seen in the urethra, they must be removed and reinserted under ultrasound guidance. The cystoscope is then advanced into the bladder, and a punch suprapubic cystostomy tube can be placed under direct visualization. The scope is then brought back to the area of the external sphincter, and a thermocouple device can be placed through the perineal skin and into the sphincter. The placement of the temperature probe can be checked using both the cystoscope and a transrectal ultrasound. It is the authors' experience that the use of the external sphincter probe has dramatically

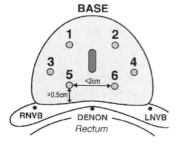

Figure 9.1 Diagram of the prostate showing the position of the six probes.

reduced the incidence of urinary incontinence in the patients following cryotherapy. Finally, the cystoscope can be passed into the bladder again, and a glide wire is inserted through the scope. The scope is removed, and over the wire a council-tipped urethral warming device is inserted and left in the urethra. The warmer is turned on, allowing saline in the device to be warmed to 39°C. The warmer is left in the urethra during the freezing, as well as for 2 h in the recovery room.

4. *Placement of temperature monitoring devices*: Prior to freezing, several thermocouple devices are placed in and around the gland. These devices can determine the temperature at their tip and in the authors' experience, have been instrumental in improving Prostate-specific antigen (PSA) outcomes after cryotherapy. Several laboratory investigations have demonstrated that lethal temperatures are achieved at −40°C, and this can be used as an endpoint during freezing. Each temperature probe is placed under ultrasound guidance. The authors have routinely placed temperature probes adjacent to each of the two neurovascular bundles, in the prostatic apex, in Denonvilliers' space, and in the external sphincter.

Initiation of Freezing

Argon cryoprobes from the CryoCare system are placed in their respective sheaths under ultrasound guidance. The tip of each probe is positioned so that it lies adjacent to the bladder neck. The sheath is then withdrawn, leaving the cryoprobe exposed in the prostate. Once in position, each cryoprobe is turned on to −10°C, otherwise known as the "STICK" mode. This will allow argon gas to circulate in through the probe at a low flow rate, but enough so that the probe will be frozen in place. This is repeated for all cryoprobes, and performed from anterior to posterior. During this "STICK" mode, small ice balls can be visualized under ultrasound as hypoechoic shadows. Once all probes are stuck, freezing is begun by turning on the argon gas in the anterior probes. This will generate a core of central ice within the gland. The posterior probes can then be turned on, driving the ice posteriorly and outside the posterior prostatic capsule (Fig. 9.2). Temperature readings in the Denonvilliers probe will start to decrease rapidly, and freezing should continue until lethal temperatures are achieved. The leading edge of the ice ball is seen as a hyperechoic rim, and can be used to monitor the progression of the ice as it nears the anterior rectal wall. Once lethal temperatures are confirmed in this region, the argon can be turned off in these probes. The ice is now extended laterally toward the neorvascular bundles by turning on the argon in the two lateral cryoprobes. This will generate cold temperatures in the lateral aspect of the gland. Freezing should continue here until lethal temperatures are achieved in the neurovascular temperature probes. At this point, the gland is completely engulfed in ice, and no visible prostate tissue should be seen. Once this is achieved, all cryoprobes are warmed by allowing helium gas to enter the probes. Active warming continues until the gland is completely thawed. A double freeze–thaw cycle is initiated after

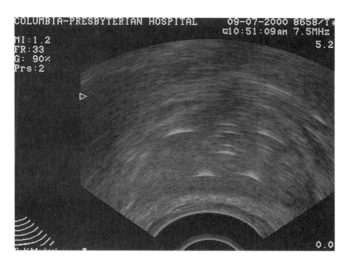

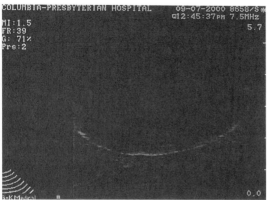

Figure 9.2 Ultrasound picture of the prostate showing the five probes (Top). Ultrasound appearance of the hyperechoic edge of the ice ball, which totally covers the prostate (Bottom).

checking the placement of all probes and thermocouples. Following completion of the second cycle, probes and thermocouples are removed, and compression is held in the perineum for several minutes. It is our experience to transfer the patient to the recovery room with the urethral warmer in place for 2 h of warming.

In summary, freezing is completed when the following criteria are met:

1. The temperatures are less than -40°C at each of the neurovascular bundles.
2. The apical temperature is less than -10°C.
3. All of the prostatic tissue appears to have frozen as visualized by ultrasound.

Postoperative Care

Patients are routinely discharged the following morning with oral antibiotics (Ciprofloxacin 500 mg bid) for 5 days. The suprapubic tube is left open for several days. Patients are instructed to clamp the tube on postoperative day 4.

ROLE OF CRYOSURGERY IN RECURRENT PROSTATE CANCER AFTER RADIATION THERAPY

Following radiation therapy (23), serum PSA levels usually start to decline (24). However, in a significant number of patients local recurrence develops (25,26). Patients with recurrent prostate cancer need restaging to rule out metastasis.

Currently, patients with clinically localized recurrent disease have limited therapeutic options. Salvage radical prostatectomy is a very technically challenging procedure and has been associated with high comorbidities and a prolonged hospital stay (27,28).

Cytotoxic chemotherapy is not curative and should be used only as a palliative treatment in the late stages (29). Additional radiation therapy is not acceptable, as these tumors are clearly radioresistant and further radiation therapy puts the patients at a higher risk of radiation-induced complications (30).

For salvage cryosurgery to become a reasonable therapeutic option, an acceptable complication rate and a prolonged disease-free survival rate compared to existing treatment options will be necessary.

Radiation therapy

1. Causes periurethral fibrosis and functional impairment, such that the effect of further local radiation therapy results in a high rate of incontinence.
2. Impedes the normal degradation of necrotic tissue in the prostatic urethra, which would contribute to bladder outlet obstruction after the cryosurgery (31).

In our experience in a series of 38 patients, we found urinary incontinence to be present in only 7.9% of the patients (Table 9.1)

This reduction in incontinence rates over previously published reports is likely due to our ability to monitor the temperature within the external sphincter.

When the temperature readings within the sphincter reach values below 0°C, the ice ball can be thawed, thus preventing damage to the area and allowing the patient to remain continent.

Moreover in our series, we did not experience any rectal fistula. This may be attributed to improvements in ultrasound technology and the placement of a temperature monitor probe in Denonvilliers' space. The position of the devices needs to be confirmed and rechecked before and after each freeze–thaw cycle.

In addition to thermocouples, we believe that continuous warming of the urethra has helped lower the morbidity of this procedure in the modern era of

Table 9.1 Complications After Cryosurgery

Complication	Number (percentage)
Incontinence	3 (7.9)
UTI[a]	1 (2.6)
Hematuria	3 (7.9)
Obstruction	0 (0)
Perineal/rectal pain	15 (39.5)
Urethral sloughing	0 (0)
Rectal fistula	0 (0)
Swelling	4 (10.5)

[a]UTI, urinary tract infection.

cryosurgery. The urethral warming system was approved by the FDA, in an attempt to maintain the integrity of the urethral mucosa and thus prevent urethral sloughing during the freezing cycle. In our study, we left the warmer in the urethra during the freezing and for an additional 2 h postoperatively. This innovation effected a major improvement in the incidence of urethral sloughing and obstruction.

The potential downside of a urethral warming system is that periurethral cancers can be left behind. Although this is theoretically possible, it is our belief that the benefits of a warming system outweigh the risks, especially in the radiated patient.

Compared to previously published studies of different treatment modalities for patients with recurrent prostate cancer after radiation therapy, we have favorable complication rates (Table 9.2). In our study the biochemical recurrence-free survival calculated from Kaplan–Meier curves was 86% at 12 months and 74% at 24 months (Fig. 9.3).

Table 9.2 Comparison of Complications of Different Treatment Options for Radioresistant Prostate Cancer Patients

Study	Type	No. of patients	INC (%)	Obstruction (%)	Rectal injury (%)	US (%)	BR (%)
Ahlering et al. (32)	RP	11	64	NA	NA	NA	NA
Rogers et al. (33)	RP	40	58	NA	15	2.5	75
Lee et al. (34)	Cryo	46	9	NA	8.7	NA	53
Amling et al. (35)	RP	108	23	NA	6	NA	74
Miller et al. (36)	Cryo	33	9	4	0	5.1	40
This study	Cryo	38	7.9	0	0	0	74

Note: RP, radical prostatectomy; Cryo, cryosurgery; NA, not available; INC, incontinence; US, urethral sloughing; BR, biochemical recurrence.

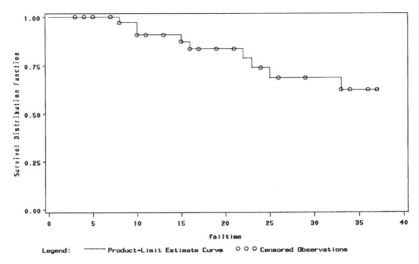

Figure 9.3 Biochemical recurrence for patients was defined as PSA rise of 0.3 ng/mL or more above their PSA nadir.

ROLE OF CRYOSURGERY IN CLINICALLY LOCALIZED PROSTATE CANCER

The treatment of localized prostate cancer is still controversial; the most common approaches are radical prostatectomy, radiation therapy, and watchful waiting, and there are specific patients who are ideal for each approach. It is difficult to answer the question of whether there is a role for cryosurgery or not without considering the relative advantage and complications of using other therapies.

Localized prostate cancer is a slowly progressing disease and untreated patients may live for many years before symptoms of bone metastasis develop and death occurs. For this reason and despite adequate amount of data about all therapeutic alternatives, it is difficult to have a standard approach that can be applied for all patients with localized prostate cancer. Furthermore, young healthy patients with localized disease should be offered the treatment with the fewest comorbidities and the quality of life following any treatment modality, efficacy, convenience of administration, and tolerance by patients should be addressed.

Watchful waiting is a conservative management for localized prostate cancer, which implies that no therapy is given until the patient becomes symptomatic from locally advanced or metastatic disease (obstruction, bone metastasis). This treatment option could be offered to older age patients >70 years, patients with low-stage and low-grade local disease and life expectancy <10 years (37).

Historically, cancer prostate is incidentally discovered in 10–20% of patients undergoing simple prostatectomy (38). It has been proven that these cancers progress in only 10–25% of patients within 10 years. The argument that supports watchful waiting is the morbidity of aggressive radical treatment, especially in younger patients, and no evidence has shown that early aggressive treatment of cancer prostate has reduced mortality. In contrast, Aus et al. (39) have reviewed 514 men who underwent watchful waiting and found hat 63% of them died of metastatic disease. The concept of watchful waiting is still uncertain and most urologists continue to recommend active treatment.

BRACHYTHERAPY

Ragde et al. (40) reported a subset of patients (stages T1–T2, Gleason score <7) who underwent interstitial radiotherapy at 7 and 10 years, 79% and 60%, respectively, with PSA <0.5 ng/mL. This rate was lower than that for patients who underwent radical prostatectomy at the same institution 98%, and much lower than for patients (stages T1–T3a, with Gleason score of ≥7), 76%, who underwent combined interstitial radiotherapy and external beam radiotherapy. Talcott et al. (41) studied a series of patients who underwent brachytherapy with three-dimensional conformal radiotherapy. He reported that 14% of them had rectal urgency, 6% had rectal bleeding, 44% leaked urine, and 18% wore pads.

In this context, it seems evident that offering a simpler alternative therapy is justified, as the previously mentioned cryosurgery protocol involves percutaneous insertion of the cryoprobes with TRUS monitoring of the freezing process. A significant number of patients who underwent cryosurgery can sustain undetectable PSA for durable periods of time.

At 3 months following cryosurgery, undetectable PSA values can be achieved in 28–85% of patients (42,43). This wide variation is most probably due to differences in patients selection and differences in surgical techniques. Cryosurgery is associated with persistence of carcinoma at 3 months in 5–18% of patients (42). This compares favorably with the reported data following external beam radiotherapy, in which positive biopsy results range between 30% and 100% (44). The most common reason for persistence of carcinoma after cryosurgery is most likely technical, due to difficulties in determining the effective probe placement, number of probes to be used, or number of freeze–thaw cycles.

Moreover, positive biopsy following cryosurgery in patients with T3 disease is reported to be <30% (43). This also compares favorably with the reported data following external beam radiotherapy that ranged between 30% and 100% (44). Long et al. (45) reported that 84% of prostate biopsies were negative after cryosurgery and 59% of the positive biopsies were present out of the treated field and biochemical recurrence-free survival at 42 months, defined as PSA <0.3, was 59% (51). Thus, and from the preceding data, it seems possible to ablate the entire prostate gland after percutaneous cryosurgical ablation of the prostate.

Especially since brachytherapy did not eliminate all cancer cells as well as radical prostatectomy, even in the most experienced hand, seed implants may leave regions of the prostate undertreated as previously mentioned.

Table 9.3   Reported Complication Rates (%) After Cryoablation of the Prostate

Study	No. of patients	INC	Obstruction	Prostatorectal fistula	Urethral strictures	Pain	UTI
Cox et al. (46)	63	27	29	3	3	11	3
Coogan et al. (47)	95	3.5	6	1	1	1	0
Sosa et al. (48)	1467	11	6.8	1.4	5	9.4	2
Shinohara et al. (49)	102	15	23	1	NR	3	3
Patel et al. (50)	169	21	7	7	7	NR	1
Saliken et al. (51)	71	3	4	0	0	NR	1

Note: INC, incontinence; UTI, urinary tract injection; NR, nonradiated.

COMPLICATIONS OF CRYOSURGERY

Previous radiation exposure appears to confer an increased risk of cryosurgery related complications. Among nonradiated patients incontinence is rare, and the most common complications noted are perineal pain and obstruction/urethral stricture in a minority of patients (Table 9.3).

REFERENCES

1. Corral DA, Pisters LL, von Eschenbach AC. Treatment options for localized recurrence of prostate cancer following radiation therapy. Urol Clin North Am 1996; 23:677–684.
2. Ghafar MA, Johnson CW, De la Taille A, Benson MC, Bagiella E, Fatal M, Olsson CA, Katz AE. Salvage cryotherapy using an argon based system for prostate cancer locally recurrent after radiation therapy: the Columbia experience. J Urol 2001; 166:1333–1338.
3. Miller RJ, Cohen JK, Shuman B, Merlotti LA. Percutaneous, transperineal cryosurgery of the prostate as salvage therapy for post radiation recurrence of adenocarcinoma. Cancer 1996; 77:1510–1514.
4. Gage AA. History of cryosurgery. Semin Surg Oncol 1998; 14:99–109.
5. Gage AA. Cryosurgery in the treatment of cancer. Surg Gynecol Obstet 1992; 74:73–92.
6. Chang Z, Finkelstein JJ, Ma H, Baust J. Development of a high-performance multiprobe cryosurgical device. Biomed Instrum Technol 1994; 28:383–390.
7. Green NA. Cryosurgery of the prostate gland in the unfit subject. Br J Urol 1970; 42:10–20.
8. Jordan WP Jr, Walker D, Miller GH Jr, Drylie DM. Cryotherapy of benign and neoplastic tumors of the prostate. Surg Gynecol Obstet 1967; 125:1265–1268.
9. Addonizio JC. Another look at cryoprostatectomy. Cryobiology 1982; 19:223–227.
10. Loening S, Lubaroff D. Cryosurgery and immunotherapy for prostatic cancer. Urol Clin North Am 1984; 11:327–336.

11. Wieder J, Schmidt JD, Casola G, vanSonnenberg E, Stainken BF, Parsons CL. Transrectal ultrasound-guided transperineal cryoablation in the treatment of prostate carcinoma: preliminary results. J Urol 1995; 154:435–441.
12. Onik G, Porterfield B, Rubinsky B, Cohen J. Percutaneous transperineal prostate cryosurgery using transrectal ultrasound guidance: animal model. Urology 1991; 37:277–281.
13. Onik GM, Cohen JK, Reyes GD, Rubinsky B, Chang Z, Baust J. Transrectal ultrasound-guided percutaneous radical cryosurgical ablation of the prostate. Cancer 1993; 15:1291–1299.
14. Onik G, Porterfield B, Rubinsky B, Cohen J. Percutaneous transperineal prostate cryosurgery using transrectal ultrasound guidance: animal model. Urology 1991; 37:277–281.
15. Mazur P. The role of intracellular freezing in the death of cells cooled at supraoptimal rates. Cryobiology 1977; 14:251–272.
16. Mazur P. Freezing of living cells: mechanisms and implications. Am J Physiol 1984; 247:C125–C142.
17. Gage AA, Baust J. Mechanisms of tissue injury in cryosurgery. Cryobiology 1998; 37:171–186.
18. Gill IS, Novick AC. Renal cryosurgery. Urology 1999; 54:215–219.
19. Falconieri G, Lugnani F, Zanconati F, Signoretto D, Di Bonito L. Histopathology of the frozen prostate. The microscopic bases of prostatic carcinoma cryoablation. Pathol Res Pract 1996; 192:579–587.
20. Derakhshani P, Neubauer S, Braun M et al. Cryoablation of localized prostate cancer. Experience in 48 cases, PSA and biopsy results. Eur Urol 1998; 34:181–187.
21. Kozlowski JM, Grayhack IT. Carcinoma of the prostate. In: Gillenwater JY, Grayhack JT, Howards SS, Duckett JW, eds. Adult and Pediatric Urology. 2nd ed. St. Louis: Mosby-Year Book, 1991.
22. Onik GM, Cohen JK, Reyes GD et al. Transrectal ultrasound-guided percutaneous radical cryosurgical ablation of the prostate. Cancer 1993; 72:1291–1299.
23. Pisters LL, von Eschenbach AC et al. The efficacy and complications of salvage cryotherapy of the prostate. J Urol 1997; 157:921–925.
24. Goad JR, Chang SJ, Ohori M, Scardino PT. PSA after definitive radiotherapy for clinically localized prostate cancer. Urol Clin North Am 1993; 20:727–736.
25. Kabalin JN, Hodge KK, McNeal JE et al. Identification of residual cancer in the prostate following radiation therapy: role of transrectal ultrasound guided biopsy and prostate specific antigen. J Urol 1998; 142:326–331.
26. Crook J, Robertson S, Esche B. Proliferative cell nuclear antigen in postradiotherapy prostate biopsies. Int J Radiat Oncol Biol Phys 1994; 30:303–308.
27. Shrader-Bogen CL, Kjellberg JL et al. Quality of life and treatment outcomes: prostate carcinoma patients' perspectives after prostatectomy or radiation therapy. Cancer 1997; 79:1977–1986.
28. Litwin MS, Hays RD, Fink A et al. Quality-of-life outcomes in men treated for localized prostate cancer. J Am Med Assoc 1995; 273:129–135.
29. Chatelain C. Adjuvant cytotoxic chemotherapy in association with radical surgery or radical radiation treatment in presumably localized prostatic cancer. Acta Oncol 1991; 30:259–262.
30. Cumes DM, Goffinet DR, Martinez A, Stamey TA. Complication of 125 iodine implantation and pelvic lymphadenectomy for prostatic cancer with special reference

to patients who had failed external beam therapy as their initial mode of therapy. J Urol 1981; 126:620–622.

31. Bales GT, Williams MJ, Sinner M, Thisted RA, Chodak GW. Short-term outcomes after cryosurgical ablation of the prostate in men with recurrent prostate carcinoma following radiation therapy. Urology 1995; 46:676–680.

32. Ahlering TE, Lieskovsky G, Skinner DG. Salvage surgery plus androgen deprivation for radioresistant prostatic adenocarcinoma. J Urol 1992; 147:900–902.

33. Rogers E, Ohori M, Kassabian VS, Wheeler TM, Scardino PT. Salvage radical prostatectomy: outcome measured by serum prostate specific antigen levels. J Urol 1995; 153:104–110.

34. Lee F, Bahn DK, McHugh TA, Kumar AA et al. Cryosurgery of prostate cancer. Use of adjuvant hormonal therapy and temperature monitoring—a one year follow-up. Anticancer Res 1997; 17:1511–1515.

35. Amling CL, Lerner SE, Martin SK, Slezak JM, Blute ML, Zincke H. Deoxyribonucleic acid ploidy and serum prostate specific antigen predict outcome following salvage prostatectomy for radiation refractory prostate cancer. J Urol 1999; 161:857–862.

36. Miller RJ, Cohen JK, Shuman B, Merlotti LA. Percutaneous, transperineal cryosurgery of the prostate as salvage therapy for post radiation recurrence of adenocarcinoma. Cancer 1996; 77:1510–1514.

37. Drachenberg DE. Treatment of prostate cancer: watchful waiting, radical prostatectomy, and cryoablation. Semin Surg Oncol 2000; 18:37–44.

38. Matzkin H, Patel JP, Altwein JE, Soloway MS. Stage T1A carcinoma of prostate. Urology 1994; 43:11–21.

39. Aus G, Hugosson J, Norlen L. Long-term survival and mortality in prostate cancer treated with noncurative intent. J Urol 1995; 154:460–465.

40. Ragde H, Blasko JC, Grimm PD, Kenny GM, Sylvester JE, Hoak DC, Landin K, Cavanagh W. Interstitial iodine-125 radiation without adjuvant therapy in the treatment of clinically localized prostate carcinoma. Cancer 1997; 80:442–453.

41. Talcott JA, Clark JA, Stark PC, Mitchell SP. Long-term treatment related complications of brachytherapy for early prostate cancer: a survey of patients previously treated. J Urol 2001; 166:494–499.

42. Lee F, Bahn DK, McHugh TA, Onik GM, Lee FT Jr. US-guided percutaneous cryoablation of prostate cancer. Radiology 1994; 192:769–776.

43. Miller RJ Jr, Cohen JK, Merlotti LA. Percutaneous transperineal cryosurgical ablation of the prostate for the primary treatment of clinical stage C adenocarcinoma of the prostate. Urology 1994; 44:170–174.

44. Zietman AL, Shipley WU, Willett CG. Residual disease after radical surgery or radiation therapy for prostate cancer. Clinical significance and therapeutic implications. Cancer 1993; 71:959–969.

45. Long JP, Fallick ML, LaRock DR, Rand W. Preliminary outcomes following cryosurgical ablation of the prostate in patients with clinically localized prostate carcinoma. J Urol 1998; 159:477–484.

46. Cox RL, Crawford ED. Complications of cryosurgical ablation of the prostate to treat localized adenocarcinoma of the prostate. Urology 1995; 45:932–935.

47. Coogan CL, McKiel CF. Percutaneous cryoablation of the prostate: preliminary results after 95 procedures. J Urol 1995; 54:1813–1817.

48. Sosa RE. Cryosurgical treatment of prostate cancer: a multicenter review of complications. J Urol 1996; 155:A361.

49. Shinohara K, Connolly JA, Presti JC Jr, Carroll PR. Cryosurgical treatment of localized prostate cancer (stages T1 to T4): preliminary results. J Urol 1996; 156:115–120.
50. Patel BG, Parsons CL, Bidair M, Schmidt JD. Cryoablation for carcinoma of the prostate. J Surg Oncol 1996; 63:256–264.
51. Saliken JC, Donnelly BJ, Brasher P, Ali-Ridha N, Ernst S, Robinson J. Outcome and safety of transrectal US-guided percutaneous cryotherapy for localized prostate cancer. J Vasc Interv Radiol 1999; 10:199–208.

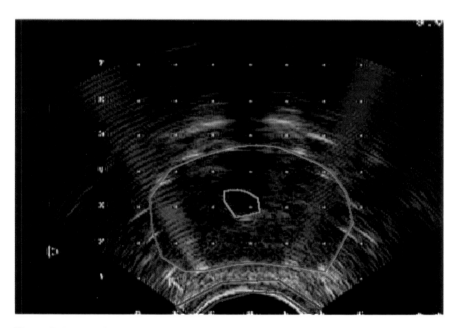

Figure 2.6 Acquired transverse prostate image (red) with peripheral needles in place is outlined on the computer using the dose planning software. The urethra (green) and anterior rectal wall (blue) are also identified in order to calculate radiation doses to these structures. (VariSeed 6.7, Varian Medical Systems, Charlottesville, VA).

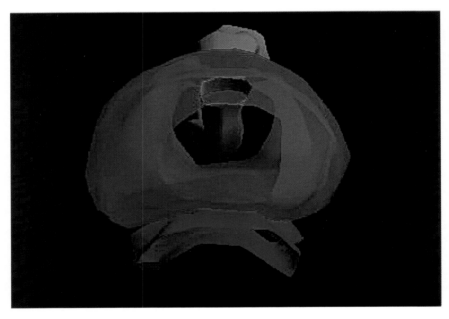

Figure 2.7 Three-dimensional reconstruction of prostate prior to seed insertion. Prostate is in red, urethra in green, and rectum in blue.

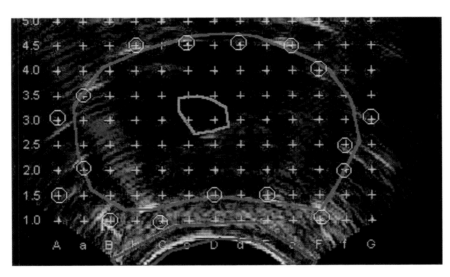

Figure 2.9 Needles are positioned first on grid point (top) and then dragged to actual position (bottom) of needle on the acquired ultrasound image.

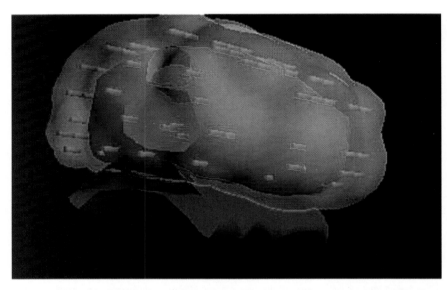

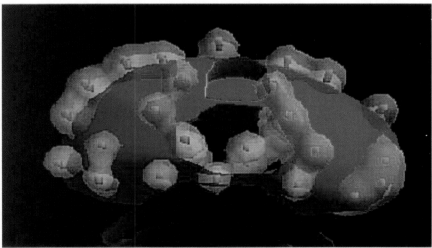

Figure 2.10 Three-dimensional image showing 140 Gy dose cloud (yellow) encompassing the prostate (top). The high-dose regions (150% of prescription) are distributed away from the urethra and center of the gland (bottom).

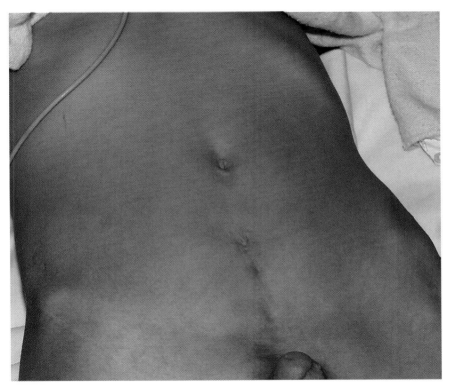

Figure 6.5 This boy with the exstrophy–epispadias complex underwent continent stoma formation and bladder neck reconstruction, and all this was accomplished through his original lower-midline incision.

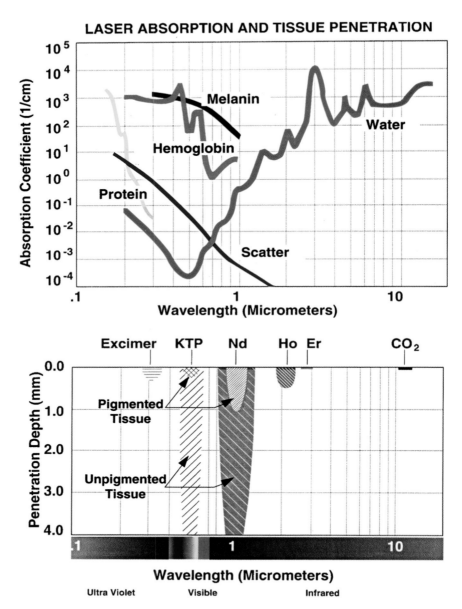

Figure 11.1 Absorption and penetration characteristics of tissue and lasers. (Reproduced with permission of Lumenis Inc.)

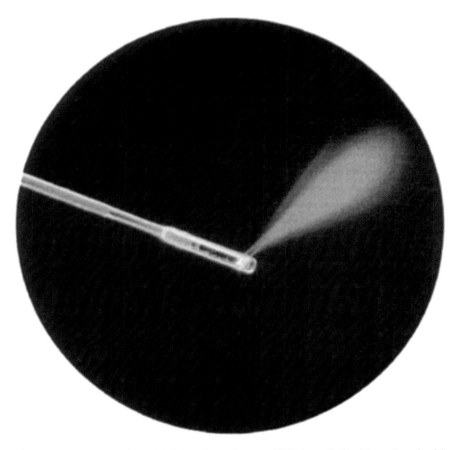

Figure 11.4 An Addstat sidefiring tip and green KTP laser light. (Reproduced with permission of Laserscope UK Ltd, UK.)

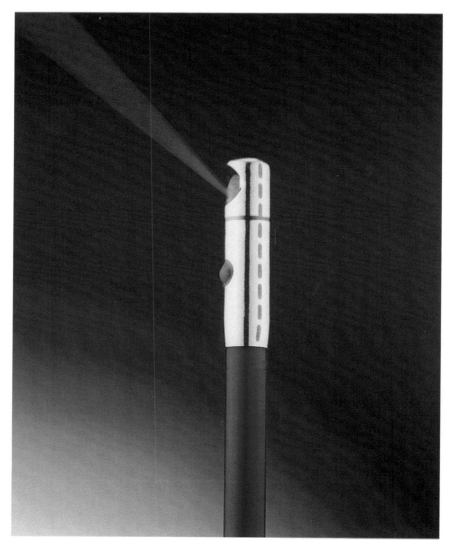

Figure 11.5 A Duotome sidelite laser fiber. (Pictures courtesy of Lumenis Inc.)

10

Use of Fibrin Glue in Urology

Udaya Kumar

University of Arkansas for Medical Sciences, Little Rock, Arkansas, USA

David M. Albala

Department of Urology and Radiology, Loyola University Stritch School of Medicine, Maywood, Illinois, USA

The search for an ideal tissue adhesive may date back 4000 years (1). The perfect tissue glue would find tremendous applications ranging from simple wound closure to achieving hemostasis. Such an agent would not only improve results of surgery but would also reduce costs by improving morbidity and mortality.

There are several requisites for such an ideal agent. First of all, the agent has to be safe and biodegradable. It should be effective in a variety of clinical situations. It should be easy to use and must be inexpensive. Though several agents have been studied including cyanoacrylate, gelatin–resorcinol–formaldehyde glue, and fibrin glue, none meet all the criteria. Despite its shortcomings, fibrin glue has found several uses in a variety of surgical situations.

Fibrin sealant was first used as a hemostatic agent by Bergel (2) in 1909. It was then used as a tissue adhesive by Young and Medawar (3) in 1940 to seal nerves. In 1972 Matras et al. (4) used concentrated fibrinogen with purified Factor XIII and an antiprotease to seal nerve endings. Since then it has been widely used in a variety of clinical situations. It has been used to control diffuse bleeding from friable surgical surfaces and bleeding from suture lines, to seal air from pulmonary staple lines, to seal gastrointestinal anastomoses, to reduce the risk of leak of spinal fluid after neurosurgery, and to hold skin grafts in place. It has also been found useful in the slow delivery of drugs or growth factors to facilitate wound healing at the site of injury or surgery. In this chapter, we will confine the discussion to the use of fibrin glue in urology.

The principle employed in fibrin glue is emulation of the last steps of the coagulation cascade. Fibrin monomers are formed when fibrinogen and thrombin are combined. In the presence of Factor XIII and calcium ions, the monomers polymerize to form a stable, nonfriable fibrin clot.

As the components of fibrin glue are derived from blood, the main concern has been the potential risk of transmission of blood-borne viruses. This has been the primary reason for it being only recently licensed in the USA, despite its use in Europe for several decades. The risk of viral transmission has been considerably reduced by donor screening, viral inactivation methods, and postproduction testing. The most commonly used purification methods are pasteurization and the use of solvent detergent. These methods are effective against the major plasma-borne viruses, namely, HIV and hepatitis B and C (5). Despite its use in over one million patients in Europe, there have been no reports of HIV or hepatitis transmission. There has been a report of a single case from Japan of transmission of parvovirus causing aplastic crisis related to the use of fibrin glue (6). Nanofiltration and ultraviolet irradiation have also been advocated to reduce the risk further. In future, recombinant fibrinogen and thrombin may replace proteins purified from plasma, thereby eliminating the risk of viral transmission.

Due to the unavailability of commercial fibrin glue preparations in the USA until recently, the only source of fibrin glue was noncommercial or "home-made" preparations. Homologous or autologous plasma donations were used to purify fibrinogen by cryoprecipitation in the blood bank. The disadvantage of these home-made preparations was that the concentrations of fibrinogen vary between preparations, thereby causing variability in the strength of the resulting clot. Moreover, the fibrinogen content of the noncommercial preparations was usually much lower than that of the commercially available preparations. Maximal binding strength of fibrin glue was found to be at concentrations of 40–70 mg/mL of fibrinogen and these concentrations are unlikely to be achieved using autologous blood (7). In one study, the adhesive strength of a commercial preparation of fibrin glue [Biocol®, CRTS-Lille (LFB)] compared to an autologous preparation was 163 vs. 114 g/cm^2, respectively (8).

The fibrinogen and thrombin are delivered using a double-barreled syringe, and the two components are mixed just prior to delivery, delivering an equal quantity of each component. The mixed reagents congeal rapidly. The resulting coagulum should be left undisturbed.

USE AS A UROLOGICAL ADHESIVE

McKay et al. (9), in 1994, were the first to report the use of fibrin glue to help seal laparoscopic ureteral anastomoses in the animal model. In the porcine model, they compared open resection and suture anastomosis of the ureter with laparoscopic ureteral resection and fibrin glue anastomosis. In this study, there was leakage from one of the laparoscopically anastomosed ureters, resulting in urinoma, but all other ureters repaired with fibrin glue were patent and compared favorably with the other group in radiologic, histologic, and renal perfusion studies.

Anidjar et al. (10) carried out laparoscopic ureteral anastomosis in pigs using fibrin glue without the aid of any stay sutures. Two of their animals later died of massive urinomas despite the immediate postoperative retrograde pyelograms having shown little or no leak. It was concluded that fibrin glue by itself was inadequate as the sole anastomotic agent for ureteral anastomosis, without the aid of stay sutures.

Studies on wound healing have shown that the tensile strength of the wounds closed with fibrin glue compared favorably with those closed with conventional sutures (11). However, there are several reasons for the breakdown of anastomoses in the urinary tract. First of all, the tensile break force is based on the width of the incision to which the fibrin glue is applied. The surface area of the ureteral or renal pelvic wall that is presented for anastomosis and thereby for application of fibrin glue is relatively small compared to the skin surfaces that have been tested in most animal studies. The tensile forces acting on the ureter are likely to be different compared to those on skin surfaces and, most importantly, the urine has fibrinolytic properties owing to the presence of urokinase. Aprotonin or aminocaproic acid has been added to fibrin glue in an attempt to delay its degradation. However, the addition of such agents results in inhibition of granulation tissue, limiting their value in this setting to some extent.

In 1995, Kiilholma et al. (12) reported the use of fibrin glue (Tisseel®) in laparoscopic colposuspension. The procedure was very brief ($\sim$20 min) and simple. Out of 17 patients who underwent the procedures for types I and II stress urinary incontinence, 15 were continent immediately after surgery. At 6 months of follow-up of 12 patients, 10 continued to have excellent results, with 2 patients reporting marked improvement. Despite the short follow-up of these patients, the results are encouraging.

Barrieras et al. (13) compared fibrin glue to laser welding and sutured pyeloplasty in the porcine model. Using open surgical techniques, the investigators performed 53 pyeloplasties in 50 swine using one of three techniques. Standard sutured dismembered pyeloplasty was done in 18 ureteropelvic units. Laser welded dismembered pyeloplasty using a 50% albumin solder mixed with indocyanine green was performed in 26 ureteropelvic units and fibrin glue was used in 9 ureteropelvic units. Stay sutures were used for the laser welding and fibrin glue techniques. While laser welded pyeloplasties were initially stronger than sutured pyeloplasties, 8 of the 26 animals that underwent laser welding developed urine leak. Six of the nine animals that had the fibrin glue repair developed urinomas. None of the sutured repair group had any urinomas. Though some technical modifications improved the results of their later laser weld pyeloplasties, this technique was found to be technically challenging and its success depended on several variables. Fibrin glue was not found suitable for this type of repair by these investigators.

In 1997, Eden et al. (14) reported the results of laparoscopic pyeloplasty in eight patients. They used fibrin glue to reinforce the anastomosis after using stay sutures to hold the urothelium together. Follow-up at 1–2 years has shown satisfactory results.

Janetschek et al. (15) advocate the use of fibrin glue to reinforce the Fengerplasty repair of ureteropelvic junction obstruction. In this laparoscopic technique of nondismembered pyeloplasty, which further simplifies laparoscopic pyeloplasty, the ureteropelvic junction is incised longitudinally and sutured transversely, and the suture line is made watertight with fibrin glue.

Fibrin glue has also been used to facilitate vaso-vasal reanastomosis in the rat model and in the closure of the vesicovaginal fistula (16,17).

USE AS A HEMOSTATIC AGENT

Rassweiler et al. (18) reviewed the European experience with laparoscopic partial nephrectomy. Fifty-three patients underwent partial nephrectomy using the transperitoneal or the retroperitoneal route. Different techniques were used to achieve hemostasis including argon beam coagulation, bipolar diathermy, harmonic scalpel (Ethicon), and Rotoresect (Karl Storz). While bipolar diathermy was favored by the authors, sealing the cut surface with fibrin glue or a hemostatic gauze covered with fibrin or gelatin–resorcinol–formaldehyde glue was found to be very useful in securing hemostasis. Recent experience from San Antonio and Johns Hopkins also attest to the efficacy of fibrin glue in laparoscopic partial nephrectomy, when used in conjunction with ultrasonic shears, oxidized cellulose, and argon beam coagulators (19).

Urologists, not uncommonly, may encounter splenic injury during open or laparoscopic nephrectomy. The rates of splenectomy following open and laparoscopic nephrectomies are 4% and 0.5%, respectively, (20). While several techniques, such as compression, argon beam coagulation, oxidized cellulose, and gelatin sponges are used, such methods are often unsuccessful and frustrating. Canby-Hagino et al. (20) reported the successful use of fibrin glue for achieving hemostasis of splenic injury following open and laparoscopic splenectomy.

The absorbable fibrin adhesive bandage (AFAB) is a concentrated mixture of lyophilized fibrinogen and thrombin deposited on an absorbable Vicryl®

backing. In a recent study, Cornum et al. (21) compared the efficacy of the AFAB in achieving hemostasis following partial nephrectomy to that of conventional suture closure with Surgicel® and a placebo group. In this animal study, use of the AFAB resulted in significantly less bleeding compared to conventional suturing and placebo and shortened operating and ischemic times.

USE OF FIBRIN GLUE AS A DELIVERY VEHICLE

In 1998, Wechselberger et al. (22) demonstrated that fibrin glue could be used as a delivery vehicle for autologous urothelial cell transplantation onto a prefabricated vascularized capsule pouch in the rat model. Recently, the same investigators have advanced the technique further and have bioengineered a tissue flap for bladder wall reconstruction (23). Controlled release of antibiotics and chemotherapeutic agents may also be achieved using fibrin glue as a vehicle.

CONCLUSIONS

Fibrin glue has been shown to be safe and is biodegradable. It is effective as a hemostatic agent. As a biological adhesive, it is useful in a variety of urological applications, despite some of its limitations in urothelial anastomoses. Its potential as a delivery vehicle in bioengineering techniques is still to be explored. It is certainly a useful addition to the armamentarium of urologists in general and laparoscopic surgeons in particular.

REFERENCES

1. Saltz R, Sierra D, Feldman D, Saltz MB, Dimick A, Vasconez LO. Experimental and clinical applications of fibrin glue. Plast Reconstr Surg 1991; 88(6):1005–1015, discussion 1016–1017.
2. Bergel S. Uber wirkungen des fibrins. Dtsch Med Wochenschr 1909; 35:633.
3. Young JZ, Medawar PB. Fibrin suture of peripheral nerves. Lancet 1940; 275:126–132.
4. Matras H, Dings HP, Manoli B, et al. Zur nachtlosen interfaszikularen nerventransplantation im tierexperiment. Wien Med Wochenschr 1972; 122:517–523.
5. Radosevich M, Goubran HI, Burnouf T. Fibrin sealant: scientific rationale, production methods, properties, and current clinical use. Vox Sang 1997. 72(3):133–143.
6. Hino M, Ishiko O, Honda KI, Yamane T, Ohta K, Takubo T, Tatsumi N. Transmission of symptomatic parvovirus B19 infection by fibrin sealant used during surgery. Br J Haematol 2000; 108(1):194–195.
7. Toriumi D. Surgical tissue adhesives: host tissue response, adhesive strength and clinical performance. In: Sierra D, Saltz R, eds. Surgical Adhesives and Sealants: Current Technology and Applications. Lancaster: Technomic, 1996:61–69.
8. Burnouf-Radosevich M, Duval P, Flan B, Appourchaux P, Michalski C, Burnouf T, Huart JJ. Biological and rheological properties of a virally inactivated fibrin glue (Biocol): comparison to an autologous fibrin glue. In: Sierra D, Saltz R, eds. Surgical

Adhesives and Sealants: Current Technology and Applications. Lancaster: Technomic, 1996:71–78.

9. McKay TC, Albala DM, Gehrin BE, Castelli M. Laparoscopic ureteral reanastomosis using fibrin glue. J Urol 1994; 152(5 Pt 1):1637–1640.

10. Anidjar M, Desgrandchamps F, Martin L, Cochand-Priollet B, Cussenot O, Teillac P, Le Duc A. Laparoscopic fibrin glue ureteral anastomosis: experimental study in the porcine model. J Endourol 1996; 10(1):51–56.

11. Lontz JF, Verderamo JM, Camac J, Arikan I, Arikan D, Lemole GM. Assessment of restored tissue elasticity in prolonged in vivo animal tissue healing: comparing fibrin sealant to suturing. In: Sierra D, Saltz R, eds. Surgical Adhesives and Sealants: Current Technology and Applications. Lancaster: Technomic, 1996:79–90.

12. Kiilholma P, Haarala M, Polvi H, Makinen J, Chancellor MB. Sutureless endoscopic colposuspension with fibrin sealant. Tech Urol 1995; 1(2):81–83.

13. Barrieras D, Reddy PP, McLorie GA, Bagli D, Khoury AE, Farhat W, Lilge L, Merguerian PA. Lessons learned from laser tissue soldering and fibrin glue pyeloplasty in an in vivo porcine model. J Urol 2000; 164(3 Pt 2):1106–1110.

14. Eden CG, Sultana SR, Murray KH, Carruthers RK. Extraperitoneal laparoscopic dismembered fibrin-glued pyeloplasty: medium-term results. Br J Urol 1997; 80(3):382–389.

15. Janetschek G, Daffner P, Peschel R, Bartsch G. Laparoscopic nephron sparing surgery for small renal cell carcinoma. J Urol 1998; 159(4):1152–1155.

16. Vankemmel O, Rigot JM, Burnouf T, Mazeman E. Delayed vasal reanastomosis in rats: comparison of a microsurgical technique and a fibrin-glued procedure. Br J Urol 1996; 78(2):271–274.

17. Morita T, Tokue A. Successful endoscopic closure of radiation induced vesicovaginal fistula with fibrin glue and bovine collagen. J Urol 1999; 162(5):1689.

18. Rassweiler JJ, Abbou C, Janetschek G, Jeschke K. Laparoscopic partial nephrectomy. The European experience. Urol Clin North Am 2000; 27(4):721–736.

19. Iverson A, Harmon W, Bishoff J, Kavoussi L. Laparoscopic nephron-sparing surgery for T-1 solid renal masses: hemostasis and tumor control abstr # 84. J Urol 2001; 165(suppl 5):20.

20. Canby-Hagino ED, Morey AF, Jatoi I, Perahia B, Bishoff JT. Fibrin sealant treatment of splenic injury during open and laparoscopic left radical nephrectomy. J Urol 2000; 164(6):2004–2005.

21. Cornum RL, Morey AF, Harris R, Gresham V, Daniels R, Knight RW, Beall D, Pusateri A, Holcomb J, Macphee M. Does the absorbable fibrin adhesive bandage facilitate partial nephrectomy? J Urol 2000; 164(3 Pt 1):864–867.

22. Wechselberger G, Schoeller T, Stenzl A, Ninkovic M, Lille S, Russell RC. Fibrin glue as a delivery vehicle for autologous urothelial cell transplantation onto a prefabricated pouch. J Urol 1998; 160(2):583–586.

23. Schoeller T, Lille S, Stenzl A, Ninkovic M, Piza H, Otto A, Russell RC, Wechselberger G. Bladder reconstruction using a prevascularized capsular tissue seeded with urothelial cells. J Urol 2001; 165(3):980–985.

11

The Use of Lasers in the Treatment of Benign Prostatic Enlargement

Neil Barber and K. M. Anson

Department of Urology, St. George's Hospital, London, UK

INTRODUCTION

Transurethral resection of the prostate (TURP) has rightly gained the mantel of the "gold standard" surgical option for the treatment of bladder outflow obstruction (BOO) secondary to benign prostatic hyperplasia (BPH). However, the morbidity of the procedure has led to the search for more minimally invasive alternatives with similar efficacy but lower side-effect profiles. There has been an explosion of interest in the use of numerous forms of energy to induce thermal damage to the prostate with the hope of relieving BOO. Radio and microwaves, high-intensity focused ultrasound, and new electrosurgical appliances are discussed elsewhere in this book, but this chapter will concentrate on the use of lasers.

Over the last 10 years there have been hundreds of peer reviewed publications describing many different laser techniques using a variety of laser wavelengths. There has been an evolution in the technologies along with the techniques and many have fallen by the wayside to be replaced by newer versions supported by another band of laser enthusiasts. The first part of this chapter aims to clear the air and help in the understanding of the science behind the various technologies and techniques applied. In the second part the clinical results are reviewed critically with particular attention paid to peer reviewed randomized controlled trials comparing the procedures with the gold standard TURP.

HISTORICAL BACKGROUND

The transurethral delivery of laser energy was initially investigated in the treatment of bladder tumors in the 1970s and early1980s (1). The neodymium yttrium aluminium garnet (Nd:YAG) laser was found to cause a predictable volume of coagulative damage to the target tissue while sparing neighboring tissue (2). It was not until the late 1980s that lasers were considered in the treatment of BPH. Canine studies demonstrated that Nd:YAG laser-induced coagulation of the prostate was safe with low risk of surrounding organ damage (3). The transurethral ultrasound-guided laser-induced prostatectomy (TULIP) device was introduced a few years later (4,5). This employed a 600 μm laser fiber coupled to the Nd:YAG laser with a 90° deflecting prism down a 22 Ch urethral probe and two 7.5 MHz ultrasound transducers. Under a general anesthetic the device was passed down the urethra and the tip positioned at the bladder neck. A series of "pulls" at various radial positions within the prostate and at varying speeds and laser powers were performed under ultrasound control. These important early studies demonstrated that the Nd:YAG laser induced a bloodless, deep, coagulative necrosis within the prostate. The necrotic tissue sloughed within 30 days or so leaving a large re-epithelized cavity within the prostatic urethra at 11 or 12 weeks. Johnson et al. (6) described an alternative technique using a similar sidefire device but this time under direct endoscopic vision. The laser fiber was introduced via the instrument channel of the cystoscope and energy from a

Nd:YAG laser delivered to the prostate tissue in four positions. Other investigators pursued the interstitial route to induce laser coagulation of the prostate using principles established elsewhere in the treatment of discrete tumors within solid organs (7). Transrectal ultrasound allowed accurate guidance and placement of the laser fibers in the prostate where large areas of coagulative necrosis were produced (8). While laser coagulation of the prostate could be performed safely with minimal blood loss, the persistent side effects experienced by patients prior to resolution of the obstruction led to interest in technologies that could remove tissue immediately, thus mimicking TURP. Vaporization of the prostate occurred with direct contact of the laser fiber with the tissue and resulted in an immediate defect in the prostate and therefore a more familiar outcome to the urologist—"what you saw is what you got". As discussed later, laser vaporization superceded laser coagulation in the treatment of BPH and a number of techniques have evolved in order to achieve this. An understanding of the principles of laser–tissue interaction is vital to the understanding of these various treatment modalities.

LASER–TISSUE INTERACTIONS

Laser light has four primary interactions with tissue: absorption, scattering, reflection, and transmission. If laser light is absorbed, the energy is converted to thermal energy and the tissue is heated up. Some wavelengths are scattered widely before being absorbed resulting in the energy being dissipated into a larger volume of tissue. Reflection and transmission of laser light clearly represents a safety issue; however, in treatment of the prostate gland these two interactions are of limited importance. The volume of distribution of absorbed laser energy varies with laser wavelengths. The absorption length is the depth to which light must penetrate to be 63% absorbed. Once tissue heating occurs, the heat diffuses to adjacent tissue by conduction. Thus, both absorption length and thermal conduction determine the depth of tissue heating and therefore the effect of the laser energy on prostate tissue. Different tissue effects occur at different tissue temperatures. At 45°C tissue retracts due to macromolecular conformational changes, bond destruction, and membrane alterations. Beyond 60°C protein denaturation occurs leading to coagulation, and finally at 100°C higher tissue vaporization occurs. If vaporization is attempted at a lower power density, carbonization of tissue, charring, may result. Carbonized tissue retains heat resulting in very high and undesirable temperatures being reached superficially, thus inhibiting thermal conduction. The key to achieving tissue coagulation in a predictable manner relates to achieving tissue heating to temperatures of less than 80°C, avoiding charring and allowing efficient conduction of heat to the desired volume of tissue. Clean vaporization of tissue relies on the ability to ablate tissue away faster than heat is conducted into the underlying tissue.

LASERS USED IN PROSTATECTOMY

Neodymium:YAG Laser

The neodymium doped YAG crystal produces laser light in the near-infrared portion of the electromagnetic spectrum (1064 nm) and is invisible. This is scattered by proteins and absorbed over a large volume (like light around a street light on a foggy night) and hence can be used to produce a steady rise in intraprostatic temperature and widespread coagulative necrosis with excellent hemostasis. The energy is usually delivered with a sidefiring fiber in free beam mode (noncontact). This technique creates deep coagulation into the prostate and the amount of tissue treated is proportional to the amount of energy delivered.

Alternatively, the effect of the laser may be more localized, that is, delivered to a smaller volume of tissue, by the use of an absorbing "hot tip" fiber. The energy is absorbed by the tip and on contact with tissue, heat diffuses into the tissue by conduction (contact technique). This generally generates very high temperatures at the tissue interface resulting in vaporization of tissue with a small volume of coagulation deep to the vaporized area.

KTP (Potassium Titanyl Phosphate) Laser

Light from this laser is in the visible green portion of the spectrum (532 nm) and is generated by passing the Nd:YAG energy through a potassium titanyl phosphate (KTP) crystal resulting in a doubling of the frequency and halving of the wavelength of the original laser energy. The effects of this laser energy are similar to that of an argon laser and may reach an output power of 60 W. Its absorption length is long in water and short in hemoglobin and melanin. Thus, in the urological setting this laser energy is absorbed at the surface of prostate tissue resulting in vaporization with shallow associated coagulation providing adequate hemostasis.

Holmium:YAG Laser

The holmium:YAG (Ho:YAG) laser represents the most recent addition to the list available for use by the urologist. Light is in the near-infrared portion of the spectrum (2100 nm) and has a large absorption coefficient in water. It is delivered in a pulsed rather than a continuous mode. In prostate tissue its absorption length is short (0.4 mm) giving it excellent vaporizing ability with minimal danger of tissue damage beyond a distance of 0.5–1.0 mm. This allows the safe use of high-power outputs to produce contact vaporization of prostate tissue with excellent hemostasis due to effective yet shallow coagulation in a fashion similar to the KTP laser (Fig. 11.1).

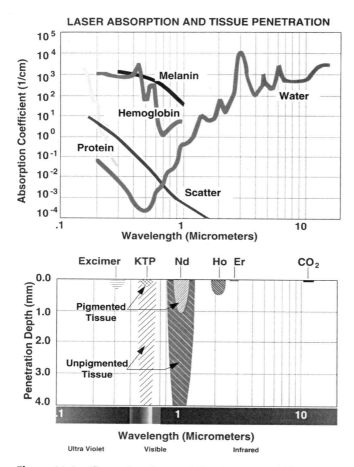

Figure 11.1 (**See color insert following page 150**) Absorption and penetration characteristics of tissue and lasers. (Reproduced with permission of Lumenis Inc.)

LASER COAGULATION OF THE PROSTATE

Free Beam, Noncontact Laser Coagulation of the Prostate

TULIP (Transurethral Ultrasound-Guided Laser-Induced Prostatectomy)

The technique described above gained popularity in the early 1990s. The balloon was dilated to two atmospheres of pressure and under ultrasound control the tip of the device was positioned at the bladder neck and withdrawn at about 1 mm/s once delivery of the 60 W Nd:YAG laser energy had begun. Animal (4) and human studies demonstrated the safety and potential efficacy of the procedure (9). The TULIP device was associated with a short hospital stay (mean stay 1.2 ± 0.5 days) and minimal side effects. In particular, only 3% described postoperative retrograde ejaculation; however, a suprapubic catheter was left in place for an average of 14 days and 20% required recatheterization. Furthermore, postoperatively, patients tended to suffer with problematic irritative symptoms (dysuria, urgency, and mild hematuria), which, as we shall see, is a feature of any technique relying on a coagulation effect. While proponents described similar efficacy in terms of symptomatic relief and quantative improvements in flow rate (10), no detailed prospective, randomized study vs. TURP has been published.

Endoscopic Laser Ablation of the Prostate

In 1991 Johnson et al. (6) described a procedure, endoscopic laser ablation of the prostate (ELAP), that involved the application of Nd:YAG energy via the Urolase^{TM} fiber down the instrument channel of a conventional cystoscope. The Urolase fiber deflected the laser energy at $90°$ to the fiber tip due to a gold-plated, solid metal alloy disk reflector tip. In human subjects, 60 W of power was delivered for 60 s at the 6, 3, 9, and 12 o'clock positions (11) and preliminary studies demonstrated the safety of the procedure with no adverse events noted. Others have described the same technique with different power settings with the aim of reducing the risks of explosions and glandular fracture and hence delivering energy more efficiently (12,13). Further modification in technique led to energy being directed with different laser protocols with ever increasing amounts of total energy delivered. Using the 40 W, 90 s, four-quadrant approach, Kabalin et al. (14) described results in 227 men over 3 years and with an average follow-up of 26 months. Eighty-seven percent of patients noticed improved quality of life with a 61% improvement in symptom scores and a 133% increase in peak flow rate. Complications from this procedure were of low incidence and included urethral strictures (1.4%) and bladder neck contractures (4.4%). Twenty-seven percent developed retrograde ejaculation and, importantly, 5.3% required reoperation within the follow-up period. Other studies have also attested to the relative bloodless nature of the procedure together with its safety in anticoagulated patients, and the use of ethanol tagged irrigant has shown that absorption of irrigant during the procedure is minimal (15). In the original study, however, overall catheterization time was long (11.4 days) and the authors commented that some patients suffered from dysuria for many weeks following the procedure and 2.6% were diagnosed with postprostatectomy prostatitis requiring antibiotic therapy. Shatzl et al. compared the morbidity of this technique with TURP, high-intensity focused ultrasound (HIFU), transurethral needle ablation (TUNA), and transurethral electrovaporization of the prostate (TUVP) (in 95 men). They concluded that there was little difference in overall morbidity in the first 6 weeks among the procedures; however, the laser procedure did seem to be associated with a greater degree of morbidity, particularly as regards dysuria and overall worry (16) (Fig. 11.2a,b).

Numerous single-arm studies have demonstrated the good outcome of non-contact laser prostatectomy as measured by uroflowmetry, postvoid residual volumes, pressure-flow studies, and symptom and quality of life scores at least in the short term. There have, however, been a relatively small number of prospective, randomized studies vs. TURP (17–21). While each study demonstrated the efficacy of noncontact laser prostatectomy in all measured parameters of outcome, TURP was generally superior across the board with a significantly shorter period of postoperative catheterization. Those treated with laser energy did, however, suffer a lower incidence of peri- and postoperative complications and had a shorter hospital stay. The latter point must be viewed with some caution as depending on local protocol this often involved readmission for trial without catheter at a later date, whereas those undergoing TURP had their catheter removed during the initial admission. In the largest and most statistically powerful study to date (CLasP), noncontact laser prostatectomy led to significantly better outcomes in terms of flow rate and symptom and quality of life scores compared to the no-treatment arm (21). In a smaller arm of the CLasP study, men in retention (either acute or chronic, defined as persistent postvoid residual volumes of greater than 300 mL), who had been excluded on this basis from the main study population, were also randomized vs. TURP. In the short term (17 months) laser prostatectomy was as effective as TURP in reducing

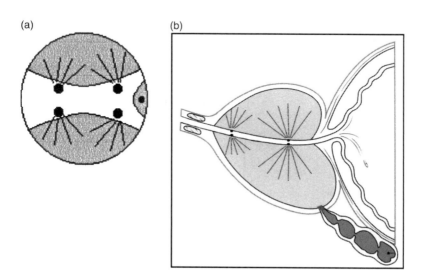

Figure 11.2 The four-quadrant approach to free beam, noncontact laser coagulation. (a) Endoscopic view treating four quadrants. (b) Lateral view treating at two spots 1–2 cm along prostatic urethra in four-quadrant manner.

both quality of life scores and postvoid residual volume measurements with fewer complications and a shorter hospital stay (half as long). However, TURP led to statistically significant better improvements in both flow rate and symptom scores with fewer treatment failures and a much shorter catheterization time (22). Interestingly, in the earliest of these few randomized studies the decrease in prostatic volume was also measured and noted to be roughly half that of TURP (17). This led to some concerns about the longevity of the clinical effect. In the only 5 year follow-up data published to date, symptomatic and dynamic variables remained statistically similar between the two groups; however, the reoperation rate in the laser arm was 40% compared to 16% in those who underwent a TURP (23).

As a result of the delay to treatment effect (i.e., the prolonged catheter time, the persistent "prostatitis-type" symptoms) and the high re-treatment rate, free beam laser coagulation of the prostate is now reserved for anticoagulated patients or those at high cardiovascular risk from the significant hemodynamic changes that can occur with TURP.

Interstitial Laser Coagulation of the Prostate

Interstitial laser coagulation of the prostate (ILP) involves the placement of laser fibers in the substance of the prostate where laser energy is applied to induce widespread prostatic coagulative necrosis. This change of approach, compared to the visual or endoscopic free beam technique described above, leaves the prostatic urothelium relatively unaffected by the thermal effects of the treatment and thus theoretically reduces postoperative voiding difficulties. There is no urethral sloughing of the tissue but instead secondary atrophy and regression of the prostatic lobes occur.

Initial animal studies using an Nd:YAG laser source and specially designed interstitial fibers demonstrated this procedure to be safe and effective, creating large volume zones of coagulation (24). The placement of the laser fibers may be under direct vision down the working channel of the cystoscope or transperineally under transrectal ultrasound scan control (Fig. 11.3).

Numerous studies using this technique [mainly using visual placement of fibers as described by Muschter and Hofstetter (25)] describe the ease and safety of the procedure and have found effective decreases in symptom scores, increases in flow rates, and reductions in prostatic volume. Muschter and Hofstetter (26) reported on the results of 239 men treated with a 1 year follow-up, describing a 76% decrease in symptom scores, a 125% increase in maximum flow rate, and a 40% decrease in prostate volume. Significantly, only 12% of patients suffered from troublesome irritative symptoms and only 7% described new retrograde ejaculation. Over that 1 year there was, however, a 10% re-treatment rate.

An alternative approach with the 830 nm diode laser has produced similar results (27,28). Others, however, have described a high incidence of troublesome

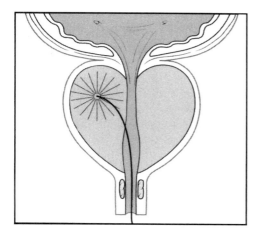

Figure 11.3 Interstitial placement of a laser fiber creates a volume of coagulation. The number and position of repeated placements determine the total treated volume of the prostate.

side effects from the procedure, including perineal pain in 72% of patients in the first two postoperative weeks (29). Newer versions of the diode laser technique aimed to destroy a controlled, reproducible, and larger volume of tissue. Short-term results show a satisfactory increase in maximum flow rate and fall in post void residual volume although, not surprisingly, the period of catheterization and incidence of postoperative irritative voiding symptoms (50% for 2–4 weeks) was increased when compared with previous studies (30).

Due to the significant edema related to any coagulative treatment there is a prolonged period of postoperative catheterization [12.8 days (28)]. However, as the prostatic urethra is relatively spared and there is no sloughing of necrotic tissue, the incidence and duration of troublesome irritative symptoms are said to be relatively low. Even so, such side effects remain common compared to other treatment modalities.

One of the problems in comparing studies employing an interstitial technique is that the procedure is highly operator dependent. The volume of coagulated tissue depends on not only the wavelength characteristics and power density of the laser but also the irradiation time and the application system. Thus, a single application can lead to a small or large volume of coagulation (31,32). Furthermore, the overall volume irradiated will depend on the number of applications and the accuracy of those applications, in that there may be varying degrees of overlap of the coagulated zones. The techniques are being refined continuously with the hope of improving the efficiency of laser delivery and may be divided into those that result in high- vs. low-volume coagulation (31,33–36). There have been a number of prospective, randomized studies comparing interstitial laser coagulation with TURP (37–41). In two studies patients were randomized to receive a TURP, ILP, or visual laser ablation of the prostate. In the smaller study ($n = 80$), at 1 year, patients in all three treatment arms were found to have sustained significant improvements in symptom scores, flow rates, and postvoid residual volumes, although these improvements were greater in the TURP arm. Only those treated with either TURP or ILP showed a significant decrease in prostatic volume (37). In the larger study of 259 patients (38), ILP was shown to produce excellent and sustainable improvements in all measured parameters; however, it was not as effective as TURP. Furthermore, a prospective randomized multicentered study ($n = 166$) employing a diode laser at 10 W of power (i.e, predominantly low-volume protocol) demonstrated similar outcome efficacy in measured parameters compared to TURP (39). In a study employing a high-volume protocol and Nd:YAG laser energy ($n = 97$), however, results at 1 year were more than comparable although there were four (vs. one) treatment failures in the laser arm (40). These results would tend to suggest that ILP is more successful if high-volume protocols are employed and this follows the evidence from animal and human studies that demonstrated larger-volume lesions at higher temperatures and greater initial power settings (24,42–46). There are few data on the long-term efficacy of ILP although it appears to be similar to the other laser coagulation techniques (ELAP), that is, ~40% at 4 years (47). There are, however, some significant advantages to this technique. It may be performed under local anesthetic, with or without intravenous sedation, thus avoiding both the need for hospitalization and the risks related to either spinal or general anesthesia (48). Thus, even high-risk patients are candidates for this procedure.

Although it is not always obvious what strategy has been employed in some studies, it is clear that generally high-volume strategies are likely to result in greater edema and firmer-texture coagulative tissue and therefore longer catheter times and a higher incidence of infections and irritative urinary symptoms or dysuria. Low-volume approaches, on the other hand, aim to provide similar outcomes in terms of symptomatic relief and improvements in dynamic variables with a lower incidence of side effects.

LASER PROSTATECTOMY BY VAPORIZATION

Laser techniques that result in removal of tissue at the time of surgery (i.e., vaporization) are of instant appeal to urologists as the surgeon not only gains the preoperative benefits of using laser energy, that is, a bloodless field, but also sees an instant response to the treatment in much the same way as in a TURP. In comparing these techniques to those based on extensive coagulation the phrase "what you see is what you get" was coined. Vaporization techniques were developed in an effort to reduce the morbidity associated with coagulative techniques while maintaining the advantage of minimal pre- and postoperative hemorrhage.

Contact Laser Vaporization of the Prostate

In order to achieve mainly tissue vaporization as opposed to coagulation, laser energy must be applied in such a manner that the vaporization rate is sufficiently fast to prevent significant conduction of heat deep into the prostate. For this to occur, the laser fiber tip needs to be in contact with the prostatic tissue in the case of the Nd:YAG laser as it should be delivered in contact mode. Different wavelengths can also be employed that do not scatter widely but are immediately absorbed within the first few millimeters of tissue (e.g., Ho:YAG/KTP lasers). Daughtry and Rohan (49) first treated prostatic hyperplasia with contact vaporization in clinical practice in 1992. Unlike previous laser fibers with 90° metal deflecting tips, which on contact would char and burn up, the Ultraline fiber had a quartz tip, an 80° angle of divergence, and a narrower beam that allowed effective tissue contact at high-power settings resulting in vaporization of prostate tissue. If held several millimeters away, coagulation would result allowing effective hemostasis. Since then other laser fibers which may be used in contact mode have been developed, including those that are end as opposed to side firing [e.g., Surgical Laser Technologies (Oaks, PA) SLT fibers with large semirigid sapphire tips].

One of the original techniques described employed the Ultraline fiber, under direct vision, Nd:YAG laser energy at a high wattage (60 W or greater) and saline irrigation. The technique involved the systematic "painting" of the prostate as the fiber was slowly withdrawn (slow-pull) from the bladder neck at a rate of 1 mm/2 s or slower, creating troughs of confluent vaporization zones by slow rotation of the fiber during each pull (50). Using this technique 71% of patients described improvement in symptoms with quantitatively significant increases in flow rate. Both these parameters were maximal at 12 months following the procedure. Most significantly, the period of catheterization was more akin to that of TURP than coagulation techniques. There were no postoperative complications and cystoscopy at 6 months revealed a well-healed prostatic fossa. Further studies using the SLT fibers have shown similar results, including objective improvements in pressure flow studies (51). While being a very slow procedure (particularly in large glands), contact laser vaporization of the prostate has, therefore, been shown to be effective. Blood loss is minimal, and as with all laser procedures, saline is used as the irrigant, the risk of TUR syndrome is avoided. Furthermore for the majority of patients postoperative catheterization time is short.

There have been only two prospective randomized studies comparing contact vaporization of the prostate and TURP. Each has demonstrated that in the short term the improvements in both subjective and objective (including formal pressure flow studies in one study) outcome measurements were as good in the laser group as for those who underwent the "gold standard" TURP (51,52). Blood loss, postoperative complications, and the onset of new retrograde ejaculation were significantly less in the laser groups. Although the mean duration of catheterization was shorter in the laser groups, the rate of recatheterization was significantly higher (28% vs. 12%). In the larger study long-term data have demonstrated the durability of outcome of contact vaporization as a technique, with no significant difference in outcome variables vs. TURP at 5 years (53); however, the re-treatment rate was higher (54).

KTP Laser Vaporization of the Prostate

The KTP laser has also been employed in vaporization of the prostate, both in a hybrid technique (discussed subsequently) and alone. The advantage of the KTP laser is its different absorption patterns by prostate tissue compared to energy from the Nd:YAG laser. KTP energy is strongly absorbed by hemoglobin and thus tissue penetration is much less. Thus, at high-power settings vaporization is achieved with only a 2 mm ring of coagulative tissue. The development of the 60 W KTP laser has led to a number of animal and human tissue studies demonstrating the safety and efficacy of KTP vaporization (55) (Fig. 11.4).

In a small single-armed study KTP laser vaporization has been shown to be effective with significant increases in flow rates and falls in symptom scores at 3 months. All of the 10 patients voided spontaneously after removal of the catheter (<24 h postoperatively) and none suffered from persistent hematuria or dysuria (56). Another similar study of 22 patients describes (57) an immediate bloodless cavity, and while 93% of the patients who had their catheter removed at 24 h voided successfully, perhaps more interestingly, 83% of the six patients who did not have a catheter postoperatively voided without complication. Clearly further studies, particularly a randomized trial vs. TURP with long-term follow-up (5 years), are required in the future to see if this really represents a possible catheterless and durable technique.

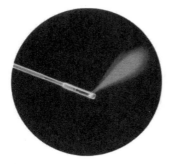

Figure 11.4   (**See color insert**) An Addstat sidefiring tip and green KTP laser light. (Reproduced with permission of Laserscope UK Ltd, UK.)

HYBRID LASER TECHNIQUES

Hybrid techniques of laser prostatectomy involve the use of one or two laser wavelengths to produce both laser vaporization and laser coagulation during the one procedure. Anson and Watson first described the true laser hybrid technique, combining the coagulative ability of the Nd:YAG laser with its vaporization properties (58). The vaporization technique could be used to provide immediate widening of the prostatic urethra by either bladder neck incisions or four-quadrant prostatotomies followed immediately by standard noncontact coagulation. The aim was to provide rapid symptomatic relief particularly in the larger prostates and decrease the period of postoperative catheterization. This technique evolved further with the combined use of KTP and Nd:YAG wavelength laser energy. A well-designed, prospective, randomized study compared standard Nd:YAG ELAP alone vs. that preceded by a bladder neck incision using KTP laser vaporization. The results demonstrated a significantly shorter period of postoperative catheterization (80% voiding at 18 h vs. 57%) in the hybrid group and indeed significantly better outcomes in terms of improvements in symptom scores and maximum flow rates at 3 months (59). However, there are results from randomized, prospective studies comparing a similar hybrid laser technique with TURP. In one the Nd:YAG laser was used to perform a "slow drag" coagulation (with some vaporization effect) prostatectomy following initial treatment with the KTP laser. Overall, while not significantly different, the outcome variables were somewhat better in the TURP arm, in line with results from nonhybrid laser coagulation prostatectomy studies (60). In the other, using a similar technique, 208 patients were randomized. At 1 year of follow-up there were no significant differences between the two groups in terms of improvements in subjective and dynamic outcome variables, and while postoperative infection rates were higher in the laser arm (29.5% vs. 5%), transfusion rates (0% vs. 5.2%) and urethral stricture rates (2.1% vs. 9.9%) were higher in the TURP arm of the study (61).

Thus, although the overall improvements in terms of clinical outcome are good, there is little in terms of long-term data, and furthermore, this technique will always be tainted by a still gradual improvement in symptoms associated with irritative symptoms and dysuria due to gradual sloughing away of necrotic tissue following coagulation.

Interestingly, one of the earliest hybrid techniques involved a standard ELAP followed by a limited TURP of the coagulated tissue (TURPETTE). The aim of this procedure was to hasten the improvement in urinary symptoms following laser prostatectomy, particularly in large prostates (>40 mL) (62). A more recent, small, but prospective, randomized study demonstrated this effect particularly in significantly reducing the dysuria and irritative symptoms of patients in the standard ELAP arm of the study in the first 3 months or so (63).

HOLMIUM:YAG LASER PROSTATECTOMY

This, the latest in the line of lasers used in the treatment of BPH, deserves its own section in this chapter. The Ho:YAG laser has also found a substantial niche in other areas of urology, particularly in the management of urinary stone (64). Other soft tissue applications in urology beyond the prostate have also been explored, including the minimally invasive treatment of urinary stricture disease, bladder tumor ablation, and resection and endopyelotomy (65). Ho:YAG laser energy can vaporize and coagulate prostate tissue and has been used alone and in a hybrid technique. The laser energy may be delivered via a range of flexible quartz fibers that are available in an end- or side-firing configuration. Following successful experiments in dogs (66), the Ho:YAG laser was initially used to vaporize prostate tissue in men. Initial studies explored the use of this laser medium in bladder neck incision to good effect, with a catheter-free day-case procedure being possible in suitable patients (67). As in the hybrid techniques described earlier, the Ho:YAG laser was used to make a bladder neck incision or channel after standard ELAP using Nd:YAG. While this did lead to a shortening of postoperative catheter times (mean of 11.6 vs. 4.1 days) in a randomized trial, recatheterization rates remained high (28%) and patients continued to complain of prolonged dysuria (68). Similar periods of postoperative catheterization were found in a single-arm study using the same technique (69). This technique rapidly evolved into a Ho:YAG-only procedure [holmium laser ablation of the prostate (HoLAP)]. Using the vaporizing properties of the laser via a side-firing dual-wavelength fiber (Duotome SideLite, Coherent Inc.) and techniques similar to the contact laser vaporizing prostatectomy described above, a TURP-like cavity could be created in a bloodless field (Fig. 11.5).

   While postoperative catheterisation times (mean of 2.6 days) and recatheterization rates (19%) fell still further, the procedure could be extremely time consuming, especially in large prostates (70). A prospective randomized study compared HoLAP with TURP describing statistically similar outcomes both in objective and subjective parameters at 1 year. Postoperative catheterization time was shorter in the laser group (mean of 1.7 vs. 2.1 days) and the incidence of retrograde ejaculation or new impotence was the same. Moreover, no patient complained of significant dysuria in either arm (71). This procedure, however, suffered the same drawbacks as other vaporization techniques, namely the time taken to effect a sufficient prostatic defect and the lack of tissue specimen. The well-known precise incisional qualities of the Ho:YAG laser demonstrated so effectively in other urological procedures including bladder neck incision and the incision of strictures led to further evolution in the technique of Ho:YAG prostatectomy. Ho:YAG laser resection of the prostate (HoLRP) is performed using a modification of the standard continuous flow resectoscope that has a circular fiber guide at the tip. Using an end-firing fiber (550 μm) Ho:YAG laser energy is employed to incise the prostate first at the 5 and 7 o'clock positions

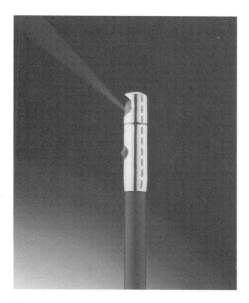

Figure 11.5   (**See color insert**) A Duotome sidelite laser fiber. (Pictures courtesy of Lumenis Inc.)

at the bladder neck, in a similar fashion to a standard bladder neck incision. At the level of the veru montanum the two incisions are united with a transverse cut and the middle lobe is undermined and lifted off the prostatic capsule in a retrograde fashion. The entire lobe is detached from the bladder neck and left in the bladder. The left lateral lobe resection starts by defining the apical margin of dissection by incising between 5 and 3 o'clock and undermining the lateral lobe a short way to the bladder neck. Additional incisions are then made at the 1 (and 11 for the right side) o'clock position in the lateral lobe starting at the bladder neck, joining the original incisions at the level of the veru. Each lateral lobe is then undermined down to the capsule in a retrograde fashion until only a small bridge remains. The bulk of the tissue is then carefully incised to create smaller chunks of tissue. Homeostasis is achieved by lifting the laser off the tissue such that the spot size is reduced, thus heating to coagulation levels only, or, in dual-wavelength machines, the Nd:YAG component may be employed for coagulative hemostasis in the standard way. The fragments of prostate tissue are then removed piecemeal using either a Toomey syringe or a modified resectoscope loop (72) (Fig. 11.6).

   A number of studies have demonstrated the efficacy of this procedure with rapid improvements in flow rates and symptom scores (73), improvements which are sustained for up to 3 years (74). It has also been shown that the procedure is relatively bloodless and that few patients in fact require postoperative irrigation (<5%). Ninety percent of patients are catheter free by 24 h (70). HoLRP has also

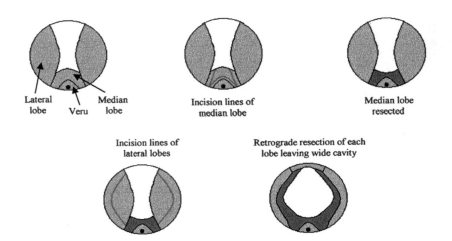

Figure 11.6   The incision lines for HoLEP.

been performed on patients in acute urinary retention with a 94% success rate
(75). A prospective, randomized study has demonstrated the advantages of
HoLRP over ELAP using the Nd:YAG laser in a standard four-quadrant technique. Those undergoing HoLRP had significantly shorter periods of catheterisation (1.4 vs. 11.6 days), a significantly lower risk of recatheterization (9% vs.
36%), and lower rates of troublesome postoperative dysuria. While objective parameters of improvement, that is, flow rates, were similar between the two groups
at 1 year, at 6 months pressure-flow studies demonstrated a definite urodynamic
advantage in the HoLRP group. Fourteen percent (vs. 0%) of the ELAP patients
required reoperation during follow-up (76). More importantly perhaps, a prospective, randomized trial has demonstrated similar outcomes in terms of both symptoms and flow rates when HoLRP was compared to TURP (71,77), and these
improvements and similarities have been shown to remain at 2 years (78).
While operating time was significantly longer in the laser arm, postoperative
catheterization time (roughly half) and hospital stay were shorter. Furthermore,
during HoLRP 64% of the resected prostate tissue is vaporized compared to
6% during TURP (79). Thus, while one of the advantages of the HoLRP is the
production of some tissue for histological examination, in fact a significant
proportion of the tissue is lost. Indeed, studies have shown that examination of
what tissue is received has revealed significant thermal damage compared to
tissue from TURP (80) and have warned that the detection of malignancy from
this tissue may be compromised (81). Preliminary preoperative transrectal
ultrasound-guided biopsies, therefore, may still be necessary for the diagnosis
of malignancy if suspected.
     The technique of HoLRP has evolved yet further with the concept of
holmium enucleation of the prostate (HoLEP). This procedure follows the

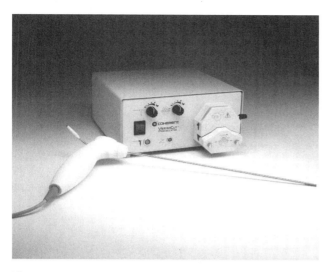

Figure 11.7 The intravesical morcellator. (Pictures courtesy of Lumenis Inc.)

principles of HoLRP; however, the median and two lateral lobes are excised intact and allowed to fall into the bladder. Thereafter, an intracavity morcellator is introduced into the bladder which allows rapid removal of tissue and has led to a significant shortening in the duration of the procedure as previously the gradual removal of the resected tissue in a piecemeal fashion after HoLRP was a significant rate limiting step (82). Morcellation has meant that larger prostates may be tackled safely (83) and the technique of HoLEP has been compared favorably with open prostatectomy for prostates over 100 g in a retrospective study, describing lower morbidity, and shorter catheterization and hospital stay in the laser patients (84) (Fig. 11.7).

CONCLUSIONS

This review of laser prostatectomy has highlighted both the benefits and the hazards of coagulative and vaporizing techniques. A GALLUP survey of American urologists compared, among many other variables, the management options chosen in the treatment of symptomatic BPH (85). In 1997, 16% fewer urologists were performing noncontact laser prostatectomy compared to 1994. Nine percent fewer were employing contact vaporization procedures and 16% fewer were employing TURPETTE-type techniques. These figures would suggest a gradual dampening of enthusiasm for either ELAP or vaporizing laser prostatectomy. One would expect these figures to have fallen even further over the last 3 years. Interestingly, however, the evolution of the high-power KTP laser noncontact vaporization technique has had notable success in early studies with, in particular, the possible benefit of the much sought after catheter-less procedure. The advent of a new pulsed delivery system, allowing higher-power densities, raises the possibility of even faster KTP laser vaporization. On the other hand, ILP has the benefits of possible application in the office setting with minimal anesthesia.

The evolution of the Ho:YAG laser prostatectomy has culminated with the HoLEP. This procedure effectively mimics the open prostatectomy where instead of a finger "sweeping" the adenoma off the prostatic capsule, laser energy is employed with the same aim. The end product is essentially the same and is associated with much less bleeding and shorter times of both catheterization and hospital stay. The introduction of the intracavity morcellator has meant a sub-stantial decrease in operating time such that it is not unreasonable to conclude that HoLEP truly represents a challenge to TURP as the gold standard. While two-third of tissue is lost during HoLRP, this figure may be somewhat less in HoLEP as less lasering is necessary. The value of examining tissue after prosta-tectomy for presumed benign disease is, however, probably less important in the modern era. The same GALLUP poll described 92% of US urologists measuring prostate-specific antigen routinely in men presenting with lower urinary tract symptoms suggestive of BOO. There is a clear policy, therefore, to detect malig-nancy if present prior to proceeding to surgical intervention. Indeed, any con-cerns regarding the loss of tissue for histology do not seem to be important for those enthusiasts of other minimally invasive techniques, for example, TUMT, TUNA, and HIFU.

But why has HoLEP or HoLRP not gained worldwide favor? The costs of lasers and attendant equipment are certainly an issue, although a recent study has demonstrated such significant savings in terms of in-patient stay that the cost of a laser is viable if 90 or so prostatectomies are being performed in the department per year (86). Furthermore, of course, there are the numerous other urological applications of a Ho:YAG laser. Concerns about the use of the intracavity morcellator, particularly regarding bladder injury, have been aired. The likely reason, however, is that unlike other laser prostatectomy techniques, HoLEP is technically demanding and requires the learning of a new skill. Nevertheless, in the longer term, as more learn the technique, the problems regarding intra-cavity morcellation are overcome, and long-term data (5 years) from prospective randomized trials are published, HoLEP may replace TURP as the gold standard treatment of symptomatic BPH.

REFERENCES

1. Mussiggang H, Katsaros W. A study of the possibilities of laser surgery. Int Urol Nephrol 1971; 3:229–243.
2. Pensel J. Dosimetry of the neodymium-YAG laser in urological applications. Eur Urol 1986; 12:17–20.

3. Kandel L, Harrison L, McCullough D, Boyce W, Woodruff RP, Dyer RB. Transurethral laser prostatectomy: creation of a technique for using the neodymium:yttrium aluminum garnet (YAG) laser in the canine model. J Urol 1986; 135:110A.
4. Assimos D, McCullough D, Woodruff R, Harrison L, Hart L, Li W. Canine transurethral laser-induced prostatectomy. J Endourol 1991; 5:145–149.
5. Roth R, Aretz H. Transurethral ultrasound guided laser-induced prostatectomy (TULIP procedure): a canine feasibility study. J Urol 1991; 146:1128–1135.
6. Johnson D, Levinson A, Greskovich F, Cromeens D, Ro J, Coistello A, Wishnow K. Transurethral laser prostatectomy using a right-angle laser delivery system. Proc SPIE 1991; 1421:36–41.
7. Steger AC, Lees WR, Walmsley K, Bown SG. Interstitial laser hyperthermia: a new approach to local destruction of tumours. Br Med J 1989; 299(6695):362–365.
8. McNicholas T, Steger A, Bown S, O'Donoghue N. Interstitial laser coagulation of the prostate: experimental studies. Proc SPIE 1991; 1421:30–35.
9. McCullough DL, Roth RA, Babayan RK, Gordon JO, Reese JH, Crawford ED, Fuselier HA, Smith JA, Murchison RJ, Kaye KW. Transurethral ultrasound-guided laser-induced prostatectomy: National Human Cooperative Study results. J Urol 1993; 150:1607–1611.
10. Schultz H, Martin W, Hoch P. Transurethral ultrasound-guided laser-induced prostatectomy: clinical outcome and data analysis. Urology 1995; 45:241–247.
11. Costello AJ, Johnson DE, Bolton DM. Laser ablation of the prostate in patients with benign prostatic hypertrophy. Br J Urol 1992; 69:603–608.
12. Cammack JT, Montamedi M, Torres JH. Endoscopic neodymium:YAG laser coagulation of the prostate: comparison of low power versus high power [abstr]. J Urol 1993:149.
13. Orihuela E, Cammack JT, Montamedi M. Randomized clinical trial comparing low power-slow heating versus high power-rapid heating noncontact neodymium:yttrium-aluminium-garnet laser regimes for the treatment of benign prostatic hyperplasia. Urology 1995; 45:783–789.
14. Kabalin JN, Bite G, Doll S. Neodymium:YAG laser coagulation prostatectomy. 3 years of experience with 227 patients. J Urol 1996; 155:181–185.
15. Cummings JM, Parra RO, Boullier JA, Crawford K, Petrofsky J, Caulfield JJ. Evaluation of fluid absorption during laser prostatectomy by breath ethanol techniques. J Urol 1995; 154:2080–2082.
16. Schatzl G, Madersbacher S, Lang T, Marberger M. The early postoperative morbidity of transurethral resection of the prostate and of 4 minimally invasive treatment alternatives. J Urol 1997; 158:105–111.
17. Sengor F, Kose O, Yucebas E, Beysel M, Erdogan K, Narter F. A comparative study of laser ablation and transurethral electroresection for benign prostatic hyperplasia: results of a 6-month follow-up. Br J Urol 1996; 78:398–400.
18. Kabalin JN, Gill HS, Bite G, Wolfe V. Comparative study of laser versus electrocautery prostatic resection: 18 month followup with complex urodynamic assessment. J Urol 1995; 153:94–98.
19. Anson K, Nawrocki J, Buckley J. A multicentre randomized prospective study of endoscopic laser ablation versus transurethral resection of the prostate. Urology 1995; 46:305–310.
20. Cowles RS, Kabalin JN, Childs S. A prospective randomized comparison of transurethral resection to visual laser ablation of the prostate for benign prostatic hyperplasia. Urology 1995; 46:155–160.

21. Donovan JL, Peters TJ, Neal DE, Brookes ST, Gujral S, Chacko KN, Wright M, Kennedy LG, Abrams P. A randomized trial comparing transurethral resection of the prostate, laser therapy and conservative treatment of men with symptoms associated with benign prostatic enlargement: the ClasP Study. J Urol 2000; 164:65–70.

22. Gujral S, Abrams P, Donovan JL, Neal DE, Brookes ST, Chacko KN, Wright MJP, Timoney AG, Peters TJ. A prospective randomized trial comparing transurethral resection of the prostate and laser therapy in men with chronic urinary retention: the ClasP Study. J Urol 2000; 164:59–64.

23. McAllister WJ, Absalom MJ, Mir K, Shivde S, Anson K, Kirby RS, Lawrence WT, Paterson PJ, Watson GM, Fowler CG. Does endoscopic laser ablation of the prostate stand the test of time? Five-year results from a multicentre randomized controlled trial of endoscopic laser ablation against transurethral resection of the prostate. Br J Urol Int 2000; 85:437–439.

24. Muschter R, Hofstetter A, Hessel S, Keiditsch E, Shneede P. Interstitial laser prostatectomy—experimental and first clinical results. J Urol 1992; 147:346A.

25. Muschter R, Hofstetter A. Technique and results of interstitial laser coagulation. World J Urol 1995; 13:109–114.

26. Muschter R, Hofstetter A. Interstitial laser therapy outcomes in benign prostatic hyperplasia. J Endourol 1995; 9:129–135.

27. Muschter R, de la Rosette JJMCH, Whitfield H, Pellerin J-P, Madersbacher S. Initial human clinical experience with diode laser interstitial treatment of BPH. Urology 1996; 48:223–228.

28. Muschter R, de la Rosette JJMCH, Whitfield H, Henkel T, Madersbacher S, Pellerin J-P, Mangin P. International multi-center study of interstitial laser coagulation of the prostate (ILC) using an 830 nm diode laser. J Urol 1996; 155(suppl):318A.

29. Daehlin L, Hedlund H. Interstitial laser coagulation in patients with lower urinary tract symptoms from benign prostatic obstruction: treatment under sedoanalgesia with pressure-flow evaluation. Br J Urol Int 1999; 84:628–636.

30. de la Rosette JMCH, Muschter R, Lopez MA, Gillatt D. Interstitial laser coagulation in the treatment of benign prostatic hyperplasia using a diode-laser system with temperature feedback. Br J Urol 1997; 80:433–438.

31. Muschter R, Perlmutter AP. The optimization of laser prostatectomy part II: other lasing techniques. Urology 1995; 440:856–861.

32. Muschter R, Hessel S, Jahnen P et al. Evaluation of different wavelengths and applications for LITT. In: Muller G, Roggan A, eds. Laser Induced Interstitial Thermotherapy. Bellingham, WA: SPIE Press, 1995:212–223.

33. Muschter R. Interstitial lasers. In: Miller PD, Eardley I, Kaplan SA, eds. Benign Prostatic Hyperplasia. Laser and Heat Therapy. London: Martin Dunitz Ltd, 2001:77–92.

34. Muschter R, Schneede P, Muller-Lisse U et al. Interstitial Nd:YAG laser therapy of the prostate: long term results and new developments. J Urol 1997; 157:42A.

35. Muschter R, Sroka R, Perlmutter AP et al. High power interstitial laser coagulation of benign prostatic hyperplasia. J Endourol 1996; 10(suppl 1):S197.

36. Muller-Lisse UG, Heuck AF, Thoma M, Muschter R, Schneede P, Weninger E, Faber S, Hofstetter A, Reiser MF. Predictability of the size of laser-induced lesions in T1-weighted MR images obtained during interstitial laser-induced thermotherapy of benign prostatic hyperplasia. J Magn Reson Imaging 1998; 8:31–39.

37. Wada S, Yoshimura R, Kyo M, Hase T, Masuda C, Watanabe Y, Ikemoto S, Kawashima H, Kishimoto T. Comparative study of transurethral laser prostatectomy

versus transurethral electroresection for benign prostatic hyperplasia. Int J Urol 2000; 7(10):373–377.

38. Pypno W, Husiatynski W. Treatment of a benign prostatic hyperplasia by Nd:YAG laser—own experience. Eur Urol 2000; 38:194–198.

39. de la Rosette JJMCH, Muschter R, Whitfield HN et al. Report of a prospective multicenter randomized study evaluating interstitial laser coagulation for BPH. J Endourol 1999; 10(suppl 1):S125.

40. Fay R, Chan SL, Kahn R et al. Initial results of a randomized study comparing interstitial laser coagulation therapy to transurethral resection of the prostate. J Urol 1997; 157(suppl):41.

41. Association Francaise d'Urologie multicenter study. Cited in: Stein BS, Altwein JE, Muschter R et al. Laser prostatectomy. In: Denis L, Griffiths K, Khoury S et al., eds. 4th International Consultation on Benign Prostatic Hyperplasia (BPH)— Proceedings 4. Plymouth: Plymbridge Distributors, 1998:212–223.

42. Lopez M, Vargas JC, Muschter R, Perlmutter AP. The size of the prostatic interstitial laser lesions can be controlled by temperature. J Urol 1997; 157:41A.

43. Henkel TO, Niedergethmann M, Alken P. Laser induced interstitial thermotherapy (LITT): in vitro and in vivo studies. J Endourol 1995; 9(suppl 1):S56.

44. Muschter R, Hessel S, Jahnen P et al. Evaluation of different wavelengths and application systems for LITT. In: Muller G, Roggan A, eds. Laser Induced Interstitial Thermotherapy. Bellingham, WA: SPIE Press 1995:212–223.

45. Muschter R, Hofstetter A, Anson K et al. Nd:YAG and diode lasers for interstitial laser coagulation of benign prostatic hyperplasia: experimental and clinical evaluation. J Urol 1995; 153:229A.

46. Muschter R, Perlmutter AP, Anson K et al. Diode lasers for interstitial laser coagulation of the prostate. In: Anderson RR, ed. Lasers in Surgery: Advanced Characterization, Therapeutics and Systems V. SPIE Proc 1995; 2395:77–82.

47. Floratos DL, Sonke GS, Francisca EAE, Kiemeney LALM, DeBruyne FMJ, de la Rosette JJMCH. Long-term follow-up of laser treatment for lower urinary tract symptoms suggestive of bladder outlet obstruction. Urology 2000; 56(4):604–609.

48. Issa MM, Ritenour C, Greenberger M, Hollabaugh R Jr, Steiner M. The prostate anaesthetic block for outpatient prostate surgery. World J Urol 1998; 16(6):378–383.

49. Daughtry JD, Rohan BA. Transurethral laser resection of the prostate. J Clin Laser Med Surg 1992; 4:269–278.

50. Narayan P, Fournier G, Indudhara R, Leidich R, Shinohara K, Ingerman A. Transurethral evaporation of prostate (TUEP) with Nd:YAG laser using a contact free beam technique. Results in 61 patients with benign prostatic hyperplasia. Urology 1994; 43:813–820.

51. Tuhkanen K, Heino A, Ala-Opas M. Contact laser prostatectomy compared to TURP in prostatic hyperplasia smaller than 40 ml. Scand J Urol Nephrol 1999; 33:31–34.

52. Keoghane SR, Cranston DW, Lawrence KC, Doll HA, Fellows GJ, Smith JC. The Oxford laser prostate trial: a randomised controlled trial of contact vaporisation of the prostate versus TURP—preliminary results. Br J Urol 1996; 77:382–385.

53. Keoghane SR, Sullivan ME, Doll HA, Kourambas J, Cranston DW. Five-year data from the Oxford laser prostatectomy trial. Br J Urol Int 2000; 86:227–228.

54. Keoghane SR, Lawrence KC, Gray AM, Doll HA, Hancock AM, Turner K, Sullivan ME, Dyar O, Cranston D. A double blind randomized controlled trial and

economic evaluation of transurethral resection vs. contact laser vaporization for benign prostatic enlargement: a 3-year follow up. Br J Urol Int 2000; 85:74–78.

55. Kuntzman RS, Malek RS, Barrett DM, Bostwick DG. High power (60 W) potassium-titanyl-phosphate laser vaporization prostatectomy in living canines and in human and canine cadavers. Urology 1997; 49:703–708.

56. Malek RS, Barrett DM, Kuntzman RS. High power potassium-titanyl-phosphate (KTP/532) laser vaporization prostatectomy: 24 hours later. Urology 1998; 51:254–256.

57. O'Boyle P, Carter A. KTP lasers. In: Miller PD, Eardley I, Kaplan SA, eds. Benign Prostatic Hyperplasia. Laser and Heat Therapy. London: Martin Dunitz Ltd, 2001:69–76.

58. Anson K, Watson G. Lasers in the treatment of benign prostatic hyperplasia. In: Puppo P, ed. Contemporary BPH Management. Bologna: Monduzzi Editore, 1993:91–101.

59. Langley SEM, Gallegos CRR, Moisey CU. A prospective randomized trial evaluating endoscopic Nd:YAG laser prostatic ablation with or without potassium titanyl phosphate (KTP) laser bladder neck incision. Br J Urol 1997; 80:880–884.

60. Shingleton WB, Terrell F, Renfroe DL, Kolski JM, Fowler JE. A randomized prospective study of laser ablation of the prostate versus transurethral resection of the prostate in men with benign prostatic hyperplasia. Urology 1999; 54:1017–1021.

61. Carter AC, Sells H, Speakman MJ, Ewings P, MacDonagh R, O'Boyle P. A prospective randomized controlled trial of hybrid laser treatment or transurethral resection of the prostate with 1-year follow-up. Br J Urol 1999; 83:254–259.

62. Sacknoff EJ. Laser prostatectomy with a TURPETTE: evolution with right angle technique. Tech Urol 1995; 1(1):11–18.

63. Suvakovic N, Hindmarsh JR. A step towards day case prostatectomy. Br J Urol 1996; 77:212–214.

64. Wolf Jr JS. Editorial: laughing all the way . . . ho, ho, holmium! J Urol 1998; 159:695.

65. Razvi HA, Chun SS, Denstedt JD, Sales JL. Soft tissue applications of the holmium: YAG laser in urology. J Endourol 1995; 9:387–390.

66. Kabalin JN. Holmium:YAG laser prostatectomy canine feasibility study. Lasers Surg Med 1995; 153:229A.

67. Cornford PA, Biyani CS, Powell CS. Transurethral incision of the prostate using the holmium:YAG laser: a catheterless procedure. J Urol 1998; 159:1229–1231.

68. Gilling PJ, Cass CB, Malcom AR, Fraudorfer MR. Combination holmium and Nd:YAG laser ablation of the prostate: initial clinical experience. J Endourol 1995; 9:151–153.

69. Chun SS, Azvi HA, Denstedt JD. Laser prostatectomy with the holmium:YAG laser. Tech Urol 1995; 1:217–221.

70. Gilling PJ, Cass CB, Cresswell MD, Malcolm AR, Fraundorfer MR. The use of the holmium laser in the treatment of benign prostatic hyperplasia. J Endourol 1996; 10:459–461.

71. Mottet N, Anidjar M, Bourdon O, Louis JF, Teillac P, Costa P, Le Duc A. Randomized comparison of transurethral electroresection and holmium:YAG vaporization for symptomatic benign prostatic hyperplasia. J Endourol 1999; 13(2):127–130.

72. Gilling PJ, Cass CB, Cresswell MD, Fraundorfer MR. Holmium laser resection of the prostate: preliminary results of a new method for the treatment of benign prostatic hyperplasia. Urology 1996; 47:48–51.

73. Chilton CP, Mundy IP, Wiseman O. Results of holmium laser resection of the prostate for benign prostatic hyperplasia. J Endourol 2000; 14(6):533–534.
74. Matsuoka K, Ida S, Tomitasu K, Shimada A, Noda S. Transurethral holmium laser resection of the prostate. J Urol 2000; 163:515–518.
75. Kabalin JN, Mackey MJ, Cresswell MD, Fraundorfer MR, Gilling PJ. Holmium:YAG laser resection of the prostate (HoLRP) for patients in urinary retention. J Endourol 1997; 11:293–295.
76. Gilling PJ, Cass BC, Malcolm A, Cresswell M, Fraundorfer MR, Kabalin JN. Holmium laser resection of the prostate versus neodymium: yttrium–aluminium–garnet visual laser ablation of the prostate: a randomized prospective comparison of two techniques for laser prostatectomy. Urology 1998; 51(4):573–577.
77. Gilling PJ, Mackey M, Cresswell M, Kennett K, Kabalin JN, Fraundorfer MR. Holmium laser versus transurethral resection of the prostate: a randomized prospective trial with 1 year follow. J Urol 1999; 162(5):1640–1644.
78. Gilling PJ, Kennett KM, Fraundorfer MR. Holmium laser resection v transurethral resection of the prostate: results of a randomized trial with 2 years of follow up. J Endourol 2000; 14(9):757–760.
79. Gilling PJ, Fraundorfer MR, Kabalin JB. Holmium:YAG laser resection of the prostate (HoLRP) vs. transurethral electrocautery resection of the prostate (TURP): a prospective randomized, urodynamics based clinical trial. J Urol 1997; 157:149A.
80. Das A, Kennett KM, Sutton T, Fraundorfer MR, Gilling PJ. Histologic effects of holmium:YAG laser resection versus transurethral resection of the prostate. J Endourol 2000; 14(5):459–462.
81. Gan E, Costello A, Slavin J, Stillwell RG. Pitfalls in the diagnosis of prostate adenocarcinoma from the holmium resection of the prostate. Tech Urol 2000; 6(3):185–188.
82. Fraundorfer MR, Gilling PJ. Holmium:YAG laser enucleation of the prostate (HoLEP) combined with mechanical morcellation: preliminary results. Eur Urol 1998; 33:69–72.
83. Gilling PJ, Kennett KM, Fraundorfer MR. Holmium laser enucleation of the prostate for glands larger than 100 g: an endourologic alternative to open prostatectomy. J Endourol 2000; 14(6):529–531.
84. Moody JA, Lingeman JE. Holmium laser enucleation for prostate adenoma greater than 100gm: comparison to open prostatectomy. J Urol 2001; 165(2):459–462.
85. Gee WF, Holtgrewe HL, Blute ML, Miles BJ, Naslund MJ, Nellans RE, O'Leary MP, Thomas R, Painter MR, Meyer JJ, Rohner TJ, Cooper TP, Blizzard R, Fenninger RB, Emmons L. 1997 American Urological Association Gallup Survey: changes in diagnosis and management of prostate cancer and benign prostatic hyperplasia, and other practice trends from 1994 to 1997. J Urol 1998; 160:1804–1807.
86. Fraundorfer MR, Gilling PJ, Kennett KM, Dunton NG. Holmium laser resection of the prostate is more cost effective than transurethral resection of the prostate: results of a randomized prospective study. Urology 2001; 57(3):454–458.

12

Stents, TUIP, Electrovaporization

Michael J. Hyman and Alexis E. Te
*Department of Urology, Weill Medical College of Cornell University,
New York, New York, USA*

Surgical interventions for bladder outlet obstruction (BOO) in men continue to expand as newer technologies are added to the armamentarium of available treatment modalities. When initially compared to the open prostatectomies, transurethral resection of the prostate (TURP) was considered the gold standard among the minimally invasive techniques for the treatment of benign prostatic hyperplasia (BPH). However, with the advent of newer alternative surgical treatment options, TURP has been considered less as a minimally invasive treatment in light of its side effects and potential complications. Indeed, while the efficacy of TURP remains unchallenged, current efforts have been directed toward finding relatively less invasive methods to surgically treat BOD with comparatively fewer potential complications. This chapter will review three of the more commonly used methods used to treat BOO, particularly that which is secondary to BPH: endoprosthetics, transurethral incision of the prostate (TUIP), and transurethral vaporization of the prostate (TVP).

ENDOPROSTHETICS

The use of catheters or tubes to stent open obstructions in both the ureters and the urethra is a familiar concept for urologists. In addition, stents have been used successfully to treat a wide range of other nonurologic conditions, such as artherosclerotic disease (1,2) and obstructive jaundice (3). It would therefore seem logical to apply these methods to the treatment of BOO secondary to BPH or other causes of obstruction such as strictures or detrusor external sphincter dyssynergia (DESD). Urethral stents are positioned in the prostatic urethra using either direct vision or fluoroscopy. Ideally, they should produce both long-term physiologic and symptomatic relief of BOO, while minimizing such complications as urinary encrustations or stent migration.

The simplest prostatic endoprosthetics are considered as first generation and include the prostatic spring or spiral as described by Fabian (4) in 1980. The current second generation includes those with self-expanding properties such as the Prostacoil (Instent, Inc., Minnesota) and the more commonly used UroLume endoprosthesis (American Medical Systems, Minnesota). Yachia et al. compared the first-generation Prostakath (Engineers and Doctors A/S, Copenhagen, Denmark) with Prostacoil in a study of 117 patients. Overall, the second-generation Prostacoil resulted in fewer encrustations, less migration, easier positioning, and longer dwell time when compared to the older Prostakath (5). Other advantages of the Prostacoil include ease of removal and its larger caliber, allowing for subsequent instrumentation.

The most widely used, commercially available, and most extensively evaluated remains the UroLume stent, which has FDA approval for the treatment of recurrent bulbar urethral strictures and prostatic obstruction secondary to BPH (see Fig. 12.1). Composed of a biomedical superalloy woven in a tubular mesh,

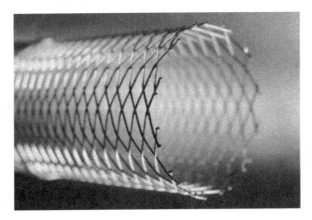

Figure 12.1   The UroLume endoprosthesis (American Medical Systems, Minnesota). A tubular self-expanding titanium intraurethral stent.

the UroLume can self-expand to a maximum diameter of 14 mm and is available in three lengths. It is positioned under direct vision with the aid of a 21F delivery tool, which contains the stent in a compressed state (see Fig. 12.2). In the USA, The North American Multicenter UroLume trial (NAMUT) evaluated 126 men, 95 of whom had moderate to severe prostatism and 31 who were in urinary retention (6). For the nonretention cohort, mean symptom score decreased from 14.3 to 5.4 ($p < 0.001$); at 24 months, peak flow rate increased from a mean of 9.1 to 13.1 mL/s ($p < 0.001$) and postvoid residual decreased from 85 to 47 mL ($p = 0.02$). For the retention group, mean symptom score, peak flow rate and postvoid residual were 4.1, 11.4 mL/s, and 46 mL, respectively. By 12 months, nearly all endoprostheses were 80–100% covered with urothelium; >50% had complete coverage.

Long-term results from the UK by Anjum et al. (7) evaluated its safety and efficacy in 62 patients treated for BOO arising from BPH. With a follow up of 5 years, day- and night-time frequencies as well as flow rates improved continuously among the surviving cohort. As this treatment is most commonly used among nonoperative candidates, over half of the cohort died during the follow-up period.

In a multicenter study in Europe, Guazzoni et al. (8) examined a modified prostatic UroLume Wallstent, which has a "less shortening" feature compared with the commercially available UroLume Wallstent. It was developed to counter placement problems associated with pronounced shortening after deployment in the commercially available stent. Although similar clinical efficacy is demonstrated in this study of 135 healthy patients, the high long-term complication rate (38%) of this modified stent has led to its abandonment. The standard UroLume stent has been shown to relieve BOO successfully in healthy patients with BPH.

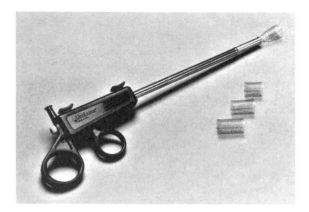

Figure 12.2 The UroLume endoprosthesis with the intraurethral delivery device. (American Medical Systems, Minnesota.)

Recently, NAMUT reported on the use of UroLume for the treatment of DESD in 160 patients with spinal cord injury. With a median follow-up of 5 years, sustained decreases in voiding pressures were maintained after stent placement and only 15% required stent removal. Overall, clinical improvement was similar when comparing men with and without prior sphincterotomy (9). Subsequent removal of the prosthesis in this cohort was evaluated in a separate study to assess the safety and ease of extraction (10). Overall, 20% of the patients required removal of the UroLume mainly due to misplacement or migration. In general, the procedure was simple with minimal complications.

Long-term results on the use of UroLume for the treatment of recurrent bulbar urethral strictures have led to FDA approval. Sertcelik et al. from Turkey evaluated 60 men with recurrent strictures in whom 65 stents were placed over a period of 9 years. After a mean follow-up of 4 years, 87% of the strictures were treated successfully (11).

TRANSURETHRAL INCISION OF THE PROSTATE

Despite the recent burgeoning of new, minimally invasive techniques to relieve BOO, TUIP was described originally in 1961 by Keitzer et al. (12). In 1973, Orandi (13) was the first to report treatment outcome and concluded that it was an alternative to TURP for younger patients with mild enlargement of the prostate. Rather than enucleating the obstructing prostate with a TURP, TUIP relies on the ability to surgically diminish the constrictive tone of the gland to relieve the obstruction. The current indications for TUIP include patients whose prostates are measured at 30 g or less by transrectal ultrasound with no median lobe present, patients with comorbidities that place them at a higher risk for postoperative complications from more invasive procedures such as TURP, and younger patients because of a lower incidence of retrograde ejaculation after TUIP (14).

One of the main attractions of TUIP over other surgical modalities is its fundamental simplicity and the ease of performing the procedure. With regard to anesthetic considerations, many have begun to use local anesthesia with good success, both in high-risk patients and in cost-sensitive medical markets (15–17). The procedure can be performed with a variety of cutting knives. However, electrosurgical loops, incising electrodes, and a variety of electro-vaporizing electrodes at a cutting current as well as vaporizing lasers are more commonly used. The goal of the procedure is to incise the prostate in one or two areas, so that the bladder neck springs apart to relieve the obstruction. The incision is made from the inside of the bladder neck down to the verumontanum and should be deep enough to penetrate the prostate tissue down to and through the prostate capsule (see Fig. 12.3). Adequate depth of the incision is indicated by visualization of fibers from the prostatic capsule or even protrusion of peri-prostatic fat. The incision(s) can be unilateral or bilateral and can be made at a variety of locations around the bladder neck. A unilateral incision is usually

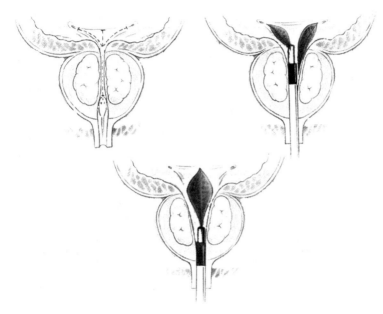

Figure 12.3   Transurethral incision of the prostate. An incision is performed proximal to the bladder neck to the level of the verumontanum utilizing a transurethral electrosurgical electrode or a vaporizing laser fiber through the prostatic capsule.

performed at the 6 o'clock position, but great care should be taken here to ensure that the rectum is not injured. Bilateral incisions are usually done at the 5 and 7 o'clock positions, although many have reported on incision(s) at multiple locations (18).

Catheters are typically removed on the first postoperative day; however, advocates of TUIP can avoid the use of catheters as a result of diminished bleeding following this modality (19).

Since TURP remains the gold standard for transurethral surgical relief of BOO, most studies continue to compare TUIP and TURP. Overall, TUIP has a reduced operating time, less blood loss, and decreased hospitalization (20,21). Riehmann et al. (22) reported a randomized, prospective comparison between the two treatments with a mean follow-up time of 34 months (range 1–82 months). With the exception of statistically less postoperative retrograde ejaculation in the TUIP cohort, there were no statistical differences found in regard to postoperative peak flow rates and symptom scores between the two groups. Patients enrolled in both arms of the study had small prostates measured at ≤20 g. Randomized comparisons for larger prostates are still lacking, and therefore the recommendations for TUIP continue to be limited to smaller glands measuring ≤30 g. Retrograde ejaculation following TURP ranges from

50% to 95% and following TUIP, is only from 0% to 37% (23,24). It has been reported that the incidence of retrograde ejaculation with TUIP is significantly lower if one incision is used instead of two, with a unilateral incision achieving comparable efficacy to bilateral incisions (25,26).

In conclusion, TUIP is an ideal, minimally invasive technique to relieve prostatic urethral obstruction. Most believe that TUIP is highly underutilized given its high efficacy to low complication ratio (20,27). Current indications are directed at patients who have smaller prostates and greater comorbidities, which would place them at higher risk for complications following a formal TURP. Additionally, men who are concerned about the development of retrograde ejaculation should be advised of its diminished incidence following TUIP in comparison to TURP. Future studies are needed to compare TUIP with newer alternative treatments for BPH such as endoprosthetics and thennoablation techniques.

TRANSURETHRAL VAPORIZATION OF THE PROSTATE

Similar to the standard TURP, TVP is an electrosurgical variation that utilizes a large surface roller electrode, which results in tissue ablation instead of resection with increased hemostasis. By combining the electrosurgical principles of electrovaporization and electrodesiccation, TVP results in simultaneous tissue desiccation to coagulate and vaporization to ablate the adenoma (Fig. 12.4).

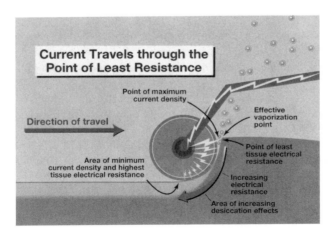

Figure 12.4   Roller electrode electrovaporization. Current travels through the point of least resistance. Current density is highest at the leading edge where fresh tissue has the least resistance. Current density is lowest at the trailing edge where desiccated tissue has the highest resistance. The leading edge vaporizes while the trailing edge desiccates and coagulates. Vaporization and desiccation are combined in one motion to remove tissue without bleeding.

The application of a more powerful electrical generator such as the ValleyLabs Force FX (ValleyLabs Inc., Boulder, CO) as well as an electrode with greater surface area such as the Circon ACMI, Vaportrode (Circon-ACMI, Stamford, CT) (Fig. 12.5) results in the greater volume of vaporized tissue that occurs in TVP. Because of its immediate coagulation of transected vessels, TVP has decreased the risk of significant fluid absorption and associated bleeding complications of the standard loop TURP. In recent years, TVP has gained wider acceptance given its similarity to the familiar loop resection, while producing fewer complications than the standard TURP. The indications for TVP are identical to patients who are candidates for TURP, with the addition of those with comorbidities that might preclude them from undergoing the latter treatment.

Specific factors that can affect the efficiency and quality of electrovaporization include generator power, electrode configuration, and surgical technique. Since electrodes used in vaporization have a much higher surface area than standard thin loops, higher power must be delivered at the point of contact to maintain the effective current density for efficient vaporization of the encounter tissue. Additionally, higher levels of tissue resistance are encountered as the tissue is desiccated, necessitating higher current. The advanced generation of generators incorporates microprocessors, which compensate with more power at higher levels of resistance. Grooved rollerbar electrodes have been shown to be superior to the standard rollerball given its ability to transmit higher current density through its grooved edges (28,29). Further advancements in electrode design include the Gyms system, which utilizes bipolar electrocautery, permitting the use of saline irrigation, and therefore eliminating TURP syndrome (30). During vaporization, the aqueous irrigating medium allows compensation for decreased vaporization efficiency due to increasing desiccation effect and changing electrode vaporization efficiency by rehydrating the tissue. In addition to adjusting tactile pressure, power level, and speed of electrode passes, time

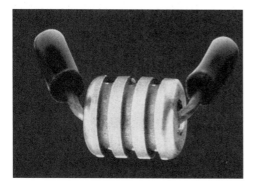

Figure 12.5 A popular grooved roller electrode for electrovaporization. (The VaporTrode® by Circon-ACMI, Stamford, CT.)

allowed for the vaporized tissue to rehydrate is a technique that makes previously vaporized tissue available for more efficient vaporization on a subsequent pass. An important caveat to the electrovaporative technique is the awareness of producing deep heat coagulation necrosis and damage at the site of contact when efficient vaporization and effective removal of tissue do not occur. This can occur when the power at the point of contact is hot enough to heat but not vaporize away tissue.

Numerous reports of TVP have demonstrated its safety and efficacy in relieving BOO (31–34). Kaplan and Te et al. described their 1 year of experience with 109 patients with a mean follow-up of 12.3 months, reporting significant improvements in American Urological Association (AUA) symptom scores and peak flow rates. Significant complications such as clot retention or stricture were less than or equal to 5% and no patient lost potency after the procedure. Randomized trials comparing TURP and TVP have indicated that both treatments appear equivalent in relieving symptoms and improving peak flow rates, although long-term follow-up is still needed (35,36). In general, the advantages of this technique over standard TURP are decreased blood loss and operating time, as well as shorter hospital stay. Although the postoperative complications with this technique are the same as that with a standard TURP, the previously discussed newer electrodes may obviate the need for hypotonic, nonionic irrigation, and thus eliminate the TURP syndrome.

In recent years, a further modification of the standard thin loop design into one that is thicker permits both vaporization and resection. One such loop is the Circon ACMI, VaporTome (Circon-ACMI, Stamford, CT) (see Fig. 12.6). Known as transurethral vaporization–resection of the prostate (TUVRP), this technique has the advantage over TVP in its ability to resect tissue, which can be sent for pathology. After randomizing 100 patients to receive either TURP or TUVRP, Kupeli et al. (37) found similar decreases in symptom score and peak flow rate. In contrast to TVP, TUVRP had a significantly lower operating time in comparison to TURP.

Kaplan and Te (38) also compared their results of TVP alone, TVPRP, and the combination of TVP and TUVRP. Their 4 years of experience at the New York Presbyterian Medical Center with 251 patients with more than 24 months of follow-up is summarized in Table 12.1. One group of patients was treated solely with electrovaporization using the VaporTrode, another group with a vaporizing loop, and a third group with a combination technique. Mean patient age was 64.7 ± 8.7 years. Of the entire group, 158 (63%) were treated with the VaporTrode (Group 1), 51 (20%) were treated with the VaporTome (Group 2), and 42 (17%) were treated with both (Group 3). Large prostate glands in Group 3 underwent a "sandwich" technique in which initial vaporization (VaporTrode) is followed by vaporizing loop resection (VaporTome), which is followed by electrovaporization for removal of residual tissue and improved hemostasis (VaporTrode). Symptomatic and peak urinary flow improvements were similar among the three groups. However, when a vaporizing loop was

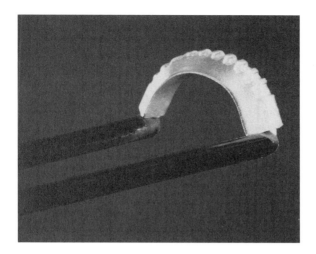

Figure 12.6 Vaporizing–resection electrode. The ideal loop would combine the advantages of roller electrovaporization to resect tissue in a coagulative manner. These loops apply known electrovaporization principles by incorporating an efficiently vaporizing leading cutting edge with a thick coagulating trailing edge. Various loops have been modified to provide a blend of efficient vaporization and desiccation. This loop (VaporTome™) produced by Circon-ACMI is one example.

used, average peak urinary flow improved by 2 mL/s. Complications are noted in Table 12.1. Hemostasis was best achieved when patients were treated with both electrovaporization and vaporizing–resection. The combination group also showed the lowest incidence of prolonged hematuria and clot retention from

Table 12.1 Four-Year New York Presbyterian Experience (8)

Technique	VaporTrode	Vaporizing loop	Combined
Symptom score			
Baseline	17.6 ± 3.6	19.4 ± 5.3	18.5 ± 4.7
6 months	5.1 ± 1.7	5.2 ± 2.6	4.6 ± 2.9
24 months	4.2 ± 1.7	—	—
Peak urinary flow (mL/s)			
Baseline	6.4 ± 3.2	7.3 ± 3.9	6.9 ± 4.5
6 months	15.9 ± 4.9	17.8 ± 7.9	17.9 ± 5.6
Complications (%)			
Prolonged hematuria	56.7	48.9	26.5
Clot retention	6.7	14.5	1.8
Dysuria	11.3	19.7	15.4
Urinary tract infection	1.8	1.7	0
Retrograde ejaculation	67.8	73.4	81.6

bleeding. Furthermore, mean catheterization time was shortest in the combination group (1.0 day) vs. Group 1 (0.8 days) and Group 2 (1.9 days). The potential improvements of combination techniques over monotherapy resection or vaporization need further evaluation. However, it is fast becoming a popular technique among many community urologists.

In conclusion, TVP is an easy modification of the standard TURP and therefore requires minimal training for the experienced resectionist. Because it uses the standard equipment already familiar and available to urologists, TVP has clear cost-cutting benefits. Preliminary follow-up data suggest that this alternative technique appears to be as effective as the gold standard TURP, while producing fewer complications or side effects. Additional advantages over TURP also include the ability to apply this technology to higher-risk patients, such as those on anticoagulation therapy. Further studies are needed to confirm the durablity of this technology.

REFERENCES

1. Bucx JJ, de Scheerder I, Beatt K, van den Brand M, Suryapranata H, de Feyter PJ, Serruys PW. The importance of adequate anticoagulation to prevent early thrombosis after stenting of stenosed venous bypass grafts. Am Heart J 1991; 121:1389–1396.
2. Zollikofer CL, Antonucci F, Pfyffer M, Redha F, Salomonowitz E, Stuckmann G, Largiader I, Marty A. Arterial stent placement with use of the Wallstent: midterm results of clinical experience. Radiology 1991; 179:449–456.
3. Foerster EC, Hoepffner N, Domscbke W. Bridging of benign choledochal stenoses by endoscopic retrograde implantation of mesh stents. Endoscopy 1991; 23:133–135.
4. Fabian KW. Der intraprostatische 'Partielle Katheter' (urologische Spirate). Urologe A 1980; 19:236–238.
5. Yachia D, Aridogan IA. Comparison between first-generation (fixed caliber) and second-generation (self-expanding, large caliber) temporary prostatic stents. Urol Int 1006; 57:165–169.
6. Oesterling JE, Kaplan SA, Epstein HB, Defalco AJ, Reddy PK, Chancellor MB. The North American experience with the UroLume endoprosthesis as a treatment for benign prostatic hyperplasia: long term results. The UroLume Study Group. Urology 1994; 44:353–362.
7. Anjum MI, Chari R, Shetty A, Keen M, Palmer JH. Long-term clinical results and quality of life after insertion of a self-expanding flexible endourethral prosthesis. Br J Urol 1997; 80:885–888.
8. Guazzoni G, Montorsi F, Coulange C, Milroy E, Pansadoro V, Rubben H, Sarramon JP, Williams G. A modified prostatic UroLume Wallstent for healthy patients with symptomatic benign prostatic hyperplasia: a European multicenter study. Urology 1994; 44:364–370.
9. Chancellor MB, Gajewski J, Ackman CF, Appell RA, Bennett J, Binard J, Boone TB, Chetner MP, Crewalk JA, Defalco A, Foote J, Green B, Juma S, Jung SY, Linsenmeyer TA, MacMillan R, Mayo M, Ozawa H, Roehrborn CG, Shenot PJ, Stone A, Vazquez A, Killorin W, Rivas DA. Long-term followup of the North

American multicenter UroLume trial for the treatment of external detrusor-sphincter dyssynergia. J Urol 1999; 161:1545–1550.

10. Gajewski JB, Chancellor MB, Ackman CF, Appell RA, Bennett J, Binard J, Boone TB, Chetner MP, Crewalk JA, Defalco A, Foote J, Green B, Juma S, Jung SY, Linsenmeyer TA, Macaluso JN Jr, Macmillan R, Mayo M, Ozawa H, Roehrborn CG, Schmidt J, Shenot PJ, Stone A, Vazwuez A, Killorin W, Rivas DA. Removal of UroLume endoprothesis: experience of the North American Study Group for detrusor-sphincter dyssynergia application. J Urol 2000; 163:773–776.
11. Kletscher BA, Oesterling JE. Prostatic stents. Current perpectives for the management of benign prostatic hyperplasia. Urol Clin North Am 1995; 22:423–430.
12. Keitzer WA, Chervantes L, Demaculang A et al. Transurethral incision of bladder neck for contracture. J Urol 1961; 36:242–244.
13. Orandi A. Transurethral incision of the prostate. J Urol 1973; 110:229–231.
14. Madsen FA, Bruskewitz RC. Transurethral incision of the prostate. Urol Clin North Am 1995; 22:369–373.
15. Irani I, Bon D, Fournier F, Dore B, Aubert J. Patient acceptability of transurethral incision of the prostate under local anesthesia. Br J Urol 1996; 78:904–906.
16. Hugosson J, Bergdahl S, Norlen L, Ortengren T. Outpatient transurethral incision of the prostate under local anesthesia: operative results, patient security and cost effectiveness. Scand J Urol Nephrol 1993; 27:381–385.
17. Orandi A. Urological endoscopic surgery under local anesthesia: a cost reducing idea. J Urol 1984; 132:1146–1150.
18. Riehman M, Bruskewitz Rc. Transurethral incision of the prostate and the bladder neck. J Androl 1991; 12:415.
19. Comford PA, Biyani CS, Brough SJ, Powell CS. Daycase transurethral incision of the prostate using the holmium. YAG laser: initial experience. Br J Urol 1997; 79:383–384.
20. Kletscher BA, Oesterling JE. Transurethral incision of the prostate: a viable alternative to transurethral resection. Semin Urol 1992; 10:265–272.
21. Soonawalla PF, Pardanani DS. Transurethral incision versus transurethral resection of the prostate: a subjective and objective analysis. Br J Urol 1992; 70:174–178.
22. Riehmann M, Knes JM, Heisey D, Madsen PO, Bruskewitz RC. Transurethral resection versus incision of the prostate: a randomized, prospective study. Urology 1995; 45:768–775.
23. Edwards LE, Bucknall TE, Pittam MR, Richardson DR, Stanek J. Transurethral resection of the prostate and bladder neck incision: a review of 700 cases. Br J Urol 1985; 57:168–171.
24. de Paula F, Donadio D, Lauretti S, Brisciani A, Florio A. Transurethral incision of prostate (TUIP) and retrograde ejaculation. Arch Ital Urol Androl 1997; 69:163–166.
25. Turner-Warwick R. A urodynamic review of bladder outlet obstruction in the male and its clinical implications. Urol Clin North Am 1979; 6:171–192.
26. Hedlund H, Ek A. Ejaculation and sexual function after endoscopic bladder neck incision. Br J Urol 1985; 57:164–167.
27. Yang Q, Abrams P, Donovan J, Mulligan S, Williams G. Transurethral resection or incision of the prostate and other therapies: a survey of treatments for benign prostatic obstruction in the UK. BJU Int 1999; 84:640–645.
28. Reis RB, Cologna AJ, Suaid HJ, Te AE, Kaplan SA. Electrovaporization of the prostate(VAP): a comparison of roller electrode configurations for resecting prostate tissue [abstr]. J Urol 1996; 155:406A.

29. Narayan P, Tewari A, Crocker B, Garzotto M, Mustafa S, Jones T, Perinchery G. Factors affecting size and configuration of electrovaporization lesions in the prostate. Urology 1996; 47:679–688.
30. Botto H, Lebret T, Barre P, Orsoni JL, Herve JM, Lugagne PM. Electrovaporization of the prostate with the Gyrus device. J Endourol 2001; 15:313–316.
31. Te AE, Kaplan SA. Transurethral Electrovaporization of the Prostate (TVP): an electrosurgical advancement of the standard TURP. Curr Surg Tech Urol 1995; 8:1–8.
32. Kaplan SA, Santarosa RP, Te AE. Transurethral electrovaporization of the prostate: one-year experience. Urology 1996; 48:876–881.
33. Te AE, Santarosa R, Kaplan SA. Electrovaporization of the prostate: electrosurgical modification of standard transurethral resection in 93 patients with benign hyperplasia. J Endourol 1997; 11:71–75.
34. Hammadeh MY, Madaan S, Hines J, Philip T. Transurethral electrovaporization of the prostate after 5 years: is it effective and durable [abstr]? 2001; 165:1220.
35. Kupeli S, Baltaci S, Soyguyr T, Aytac S, Yilmaz E, Budak M. A prospective randomized study of transurethral resection of the prostate and transurethral vaporization of the prostate as atherapeutic alternative in the management of men with BPH. Eur Urol 1998; 34:15–18.
36. Kaplan SA, Laor E, Fatal M, Te AE. Transurethral resection of the prostate versus transurethral electrovaporization of the prostate: a blinded, prospective comparative study with 1-year followup. J Urol 1998; 159:454–458.
37. Kupeli S, Yilmaz E, Soygur T, Budak M. Randomized study of transurethral resection of the prostate and combined transurethral resection and vaporization of the prostate as a therapeutic alternative in men with benign prostatic hyperplasia. J Endourol 2001; 15:317–321.
38. Nejat RJ, Ikeguchi EF, Te AE, Reis RB, Kaplan SA. Electrovaporization of the prostateutilizing the roller ball and/or vaporizing loop for the symptomatic benign prostatic hyperplasia(BPH): the 4-year Columbia experience. J Urol 1999; 161(4):391.

13

Erectile Dysfunction: Evolution from Maximally to Minimally Invasive

Judy Chun, John Kang, Aubrey Evans, and Culley C. Carson
*Division of Urologic Surgery, University of North Carolina Hospitals,
Chapel Hill, North Carolina, USA*

The association between the testes, male behavior, potency, and fertility has been recognized since man began the practice of castration to domesticate animals as early as 4000 BC. From the early 19th to the mid-20th centuries, the cause of erectile dysfunction (ED), traditionally referred to as impotence, was believed to be an endocrine imbalance. Treatments ranged from ligation of the vas deferens to promotion of endogenous male hormone production to surgical transplantation of testicular grafts from apes (1,2). Fortunately, in 1934, Lower (3) demonstrated the pituitary gonadotrophic control of the testis to elucidate the male genitourinary and reproductive physiology which curtailed these questionable treatment practices.

Further hypotheses of ED were initiated in the late 19th and early 20th centuries with a spirited debate between the "psychogenic versus organic" causes. In 1927, followers of Sigmund Freud stated that repressed sexuality was responsible for at least 95% of ED cases (4). Freud's disciples believed that transference of unresolved feelings from the oedipal stage of infant development to a new sexual partner could result in inner conflict leading to ED. Treatment involved years of psychoanalysis and resensitization of the erectile mechanism through abstinence from sexual intercourse for long periods of time. The "organic" school of thought, led by urologists, countered with elaborate descriptions of the multiple pathologies observed. These ranged from venereal disease to inflammation of the verumontanum in the posterior urethra, supposedly leading to uncontrollable urges toward sexual excess. The indulgence of this urge, either through frequent coitus or masturbation, was thought to desensitize the central erectile center and induce impotence (5). Treatment encompassed multiple procedures designed to reduce this urge.

Whether the etiology of ED was thought to originate from endocrine imbalance, or psychogenic or organic elements, unfortunately, all of the available treatments—psychoanalysis, aphrodisiacs, vasoligation, testicular grafting, forced abstinence, and desensitization—proved disappointing. The lack of viable treatment options, coupled with the anxieties surrounding taboo sexual topics, created an atmosphere where physicians rarely questioned patients about sexual function, and patients rarely sought advice on sexual concerns. This environment persisted through the early 1980s, when it was still believed that up to 90% of all ED cases had a psychogenic etiology.

Considerable advances in our understanding of erectile physiology and pathophysiology have been made, revealing the complex, multifactoral components involved in ED. The term impotence is a vague, all-encompassing definition of male sexual dysfunction, including loss of sexual drive, orgasmic or ejaculatory dysfunction, and ED (6). In 1992, the National Institute of Health Consensus Panel set out to educate health care providers and improve public awareness on aspects of human sexuality and sexual dysfunction. They defined ED as the inability to achieve or maintain an erection sufficient for satisfactory sexual function (6). Due to the negative, stigmatizing connotations associated with "impotence", the preferred terminology is more descriptive and more physiologic: vasculogenic, endocrinologic, neurogenic, psychogenic, traumatic, or iatrogenic ED.

EPIDEMIOLOGY

ED is the second most common sexual problem in men, after premature ejaculation, affecting up to 30 million men in the USA (7). Historically, the prevalence of impotence has been difficult to estimate due to the fact that it is not a life-threatening disease, and because patients are reluctant to discuss embarrassing conditions openly. The first extensive epidemiologic study on male sexual behavior in the USA was reported in 1948 by Kinsey et al. (6) They "concluded that the prevalence of ED was <1% in men younger than 30, <3% in those younger than 45, 6.7% in those 45–55, 25% in those 65, and up to 80% in those 80 years old". It is important to note that the sample size for men older than 55 years was disproportionately small. According to the Massachusetts Male Aging Study (MMAS), probably the single most useful study on male sexuality conducted from 1987 to 1989, the prevalence of impotence of all degrees is approximately 52%, a condition with wide-reaching implications (8). A more recent study from the 1992 National Health and Social Life Survey found sexual dysfunction to affect 31% of men (9). There is little or no information on the prevalence of ED in relationship to ethnicity or socioeconomic status.

RISK FACTORS

Many potential risk factors have been identified for ED, including atherosclerosis, diabetes mellitus, and tobacco. The common denominator for these risk factors, also thought to be the major cause of organic ED, is impaired vascular function. Arteriosclerosis causes vascular alterations in the penile arteries, which impede blood flow to the cavernous bodies. Several studies demonstrated a high prevalence of ED in men with vascular disease: 64% of men who suffered a myocardial infarction and 57% of men with coronary artery bypass surgery (10,11). The eight million diabetic adult men in the USA have a much higher prevalence of ED than the general population, ranging from 35% to 59% (12). Moreover, the onset of ED occurs an average of 10–15 years earlier and is the most common feature of diabetic autonomic neuropathy (13). Cigarette smoking is perhaps the most important modifiable risk factor of ED. A history of 5, 10, and 20 years of tobacco exposure are associated with 15%, 30%, and 70% incidence of arterial occlusive disease within the common penile artery, respectively (14). In the MMAS (8), among subjects with treated heart disease, the age-adjusted probability of complete ED was 56% for smokers vs. 21% for nonsmokers. Among treated hypertensive men, smokers had a 20% incidence of ED, compared to nonsmokers who were comparable to the general population at 8.5%.

As many as a quarter of ED cases may be attributable to prescription medications (15). The list is extensive and includes antidepressants, antipsychotics, diuretics, antihypertensives and other vasodilators, estrogens, progestins, and luteinizing hormone-releasing hormone agonists and antagonists (16). Of the medications listed in Table 13.1, thiazide diuretics are the most common culprits

Table 13.1   Medications Affecting Erectile Dysfunction

Diuretics	Thiazide
	Spironolactone
Antihypertensives	Methyldopa
	Clonidine
	Reserpine
	Beta-blockers
	Verapamil
Cardiac/circulatory	Gemfibrizol
	Digoxin
	Clofibrate
Tranquilizers	Phenethiazines
	Butyrophenones
Antidepressants	Tricyclic antidepressants
	Lithium
	Monoamine oxidase inhibitors
	Selective serotonin reuptake inhibitors
H2-antagonists	Cimetidine
	Ranitidine
Hormones	Estrogens
	Progesterones
	5-Alpha reductase inhibitors
	Luteinizing hormone–releasing horomone agonist
	Corticosterones
	Cyproterone acetates
Cytotoxic agents	Cyclophosphamide
	Methotrexate
Anticholinergics	Dysopyramide
	Anticonvulsants
Recreational	Alcohol
	Marijuana
	Cocaine

because of their frequent usage. The ways in which medications can cause ED are quite varied and include interference with the parasympathetic erectile mechanism, stimulation of the alpha-adrenergic vasoconstrictor tone, interference with central responses to erotic stimuli, and production of endocrine effects by affecting the dopamine inhibition of prolactin.

These advances in our understanding of ED have allowed an evolution from maximally to minimally invasive treatment options. Until three decades ago, ED was primarily treated with testosterone injections and psychotherapy. The role of androgens in the maintenance of erectile function remain poorly understood, but hormone replacement is recommended solely for ED patients with documented hypogonadism, only 3–6% of all ED cases. A new era in ED treatments began in the mid-1970s with the development of an effective penile prosthesis. Another advance occurred in the 1980s with the development of intracavernous injection of vasoactive drugs. At the end of the 1980s, vacuum therapy emerged as a third major alternative for treatment of ED. But, by far the most wide-reaching treatment was the introduction of an effective oral medication, sildenafil (Viagra), in 1998. Sildenafil, prescribed in >90% of ED cases in the USA, has been shown to treat ED successfully in a dose-dependent manner, with 69% of attempts being successful at the maximal dose of 100 mg given 60–90 min before intercourse (17). The success of this medication and its mainstream advertising campaign have initiated an unheralded awareness of ED within the general population. The rest of the chapter is dedicated to the detailed history of the maximally to minimally invasive treatments of ED (Table 13.2) and the implications associated with it.

PENILE PROSTHESIS

Maximally invasive surgical interventions were born out of necessity during the Second World War as many pilots and soldiers suffered loss of genitalia as a result of burn injuries or land mines. Generally, surgery has one of three mechanisms to restore or produce erections: (1) implant a penile device, (2) increase arterial flow to the penis, or (3) impede venous leak from the cavernosal tissues. The first major alternative to testosterone treatment for ED was the development of a penile prosthesis. In 1948, Bergman et al. (18) fashioned a new penis over an autografted rib cartilage, but the process was limited by reabsorption of the cartilage. By 1964, the insertion of acrylic rods into the penis was reported to successfully treat ED (19). These implants became common and successful until the development of silicone elastomer and the introduction of the Small-Carnion and Scott prostheses in 1973.

Two basic types of prosthesis are available: semirigid rods and inflatable cylinders. The semirigid rods can further be divided into mechanical (Omniphase, Duraphase, Dura II) and malleable [Jonas Bard, American Medical Systems (AMS) 600, AMS 650, Mentor] implants. The mechanical implants consist of two rod-like cylinders composed of a series of polysulfone segments

Table 13.2 Maximally to Minimally Invasive
Treatment for Erectile Dysfunction

Penile prostheses
  Semirigid rods
  Inflatable penile prosthesis
Arterial and venous revascularization
Vacuum constriction device
Intracavernous injection therapy
  Papaverine and phentolamine
  Alprostadil
  Moxisylyte chlorhydrate (Icavex)
  Vasoactive intestinal polypeptide (VIP)
Medicated urethral system for erections (MUSE)
Sildenafil (Viagra)
Other oral agents
  Herbal therapy
  Trazadone
  Yohimbine
  Delaquamine and phentolamine (Vasomax)
  L-Arginine
  Apomorphine (Uprima)
  Cialis and vardenafil
Gene therapy

---

that articulate in a ball and socket arrangement held together by a central cable attached to a spring (20). The malleable implants have a braided silver or stainless steel core surrounded by solid silicone. The semirigid rods were popular because they are self-contained and easy to insert. The paired rods are implanted into the twin corpora, and the user manually models the position of the rods within the penis. They provide reasonable rigidity and are very easy to manipulate. However, adjustments do not affect the width or length of the penis, and patients with a very broad penis achieve suboptimal axial rigidity for penetration. Some patient dissatisfaction comes from cosmetic concerns of the semirigid, malleable devices springing back and protruding under clothing. One of the advantages of the inflatable penile prosthesis (IPP) is that it mimics the natural penis. The inflatable implants consist of paired cylinders that can expand the girth and length of the penis using pressurized fluid for a rigid erection and be drained when not in use to obtain a flaccid, natural state. There are currently three available hydraulically inflatable penile prostheses: self-contained (AMS Dynaflex), two-piece (Mentor GFS Mark II, AMS Ambicor), and three-piece (AMS 700 CX, AMS Ultrex and Ultrex plus, Mentor Alpha-1). Composition of the inflatable cylinders ranges from a three-layer construction of inner silicone layer, middle Dacron mesh or Lycra layer, and an outer layer of silicone for AMS implants to a single layer of Bioflex for Mentor cylinders (21). In the three-piece prosthesis, nonkinked plastic tubing connects the cylinders to a fluid reservoir, surgically implanted into the extraperitoneal abdomen, and a scrotal hand pump, unlike the two-piece prosthesis where the reservoir also serves as the pump. In both of the systems, the patient needs manual dexterity and coordination to inflate the corporal cylinders by pumping fluid from the reservoir into the cylinders.

Despite the availability of less invasive alternatives for ED, the penile implant has remained in demand. About 21,000 implants were sold in the USA in 1996 (20). Overall patient satisfaction is high for both semirigid and inflatable implants. In a series of over 700 patients with an inflatable implant, overall satisfaction was 90% (22). Chiang (23) reported patient satisfaction at 86.6% at 10 years.

The most worrisome complication is prosthesis infection, $\sim 1.6\%$ for semi-rigid rods and 4.3% for IPP (24). Patients at increased risk are diabetics, immunocompromised patients, those with urinary tract bacterial colonization from indwelling catheters, and those undergoing additional procedures with the implant such as circumcision or penile straightening. Most prosthesis infections begin with bacterial seeding during surgery with normal skin flora, *Staphylococcus epidermidis*, and other gram-positive organisms. Prosthesis extrusion or erosion is most common in patients with compromised tissue or decreased genital sensation, for example, due to diabetes mellitus, spinal cord injury, or previous infections. However, overall complication rates remain low (20).

Semirigid rods are associated with fewer mechanical complications than the multicomponent IPP, lasting $\sim 6-8$ years (24). Decreased rigidity in the semi-rigid prosthesis has been reported, indicating fracture or breakage of the central wire. Because the cylinder portion of the inflatable prosthesis functions at significantly higher pressures than the rest of the components, most mechanical breakdowns occur in the cylinders as aneurysmal dilatation. Autoinflation occurs when the pressure around the reservoir pushes the fluid into the cylinders. Garber (25) reported a complication rate of 3% in 150 IPP cases, two peri-prosthetic infections, and two intraoperative and one postoperative cylinder aneurysm. Penile implants are a viable treatment option, although they are primarily utilized only after more conservative forms of therapy fail (Fig. 13.1).

ARTERIAL AND VENOUS REVASCULARIZATION

Michal et al. (26) published the first report on penile revascularization in 1972. Theoretically, microvascular arterial bypass surgery restores full erectile blood flow to the penis during sexual stimulation. Various modifications have developed with different donor arteries (inferior epigastric artery, femoral artery) to various recipients (deep dorsal vein, tunica albuginea, dorsal penile artery). Candidates for microvascular artery bypass surgery are evaluated initially by penile Doppler ultrasound to assess the blood flow in the dorsal arteries, as well as the patency and flow in the deep dorsal vein. If needed, further details

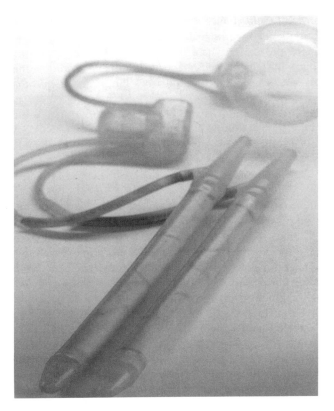

Figure 13.1   Inflatable penile prosthesis.

are mapped by pelvic angiography to identify pathology in the common iliac arteries or in the origin of the hypogastric arteries, and for visualization of the inferior epigastric arteries and the dorsal arteries prior to surgery.

Experimental series published in the past 5–10 years have used a variety of procedures with varied patient populations, indications, and techniques. Reported long-term success rates range from 25% to 80% (27,28). Unfortunately, accurate interpretation of the results is limited due to the lack of standardization. As a whole, surgery has proven efficacious only in young men with arterial insufficiency secondary to pelvic trauma (29).

The most frequently reported complication of arterial revascularization is hyperemia of the glans, occurring in 7–13% of patients (26,30). Prompt attention is needed in these patients to avoid glanular tissue loss. Other commonly reported complications include hematomas, thromboses of the vascular anastomosis, and infection. Numerous diagnostic refinements and strict patient selection criteria have not improved the outcome. Arterial revascularization is still considered an investigational procedure, and the optimal candidate is a young neurologically intact male with vasculogenic ED from trauma, not systemic disease.

The first attempts to treat veno-occlusive ED through a surgical approach were by Wooten in 1902 and Lydston in 1908. Nonetheless, penile vein ligation was not performed commonly until 1985 (31). Surgical candidates are patients with physiologic evidence of venous leakage on dynamic pharmacavernosometry and cavernosography, or patients with poor to no response to intracavernosal vasoactive agents. Surgery involves penile vein ligation or embolization to reduce the number of channels for venous outflow and therefore increases venous resistance. Unfortunately, success rates for veno-occlusive disease generally have been poor. Success rates within the first year range from 23% to 80% but consistently decrease on longer follow-up (14–77%) (29,32,33).

Complications of venous channel ligations include penile curvatures, painful erections, wound infections, skin necrosis, and proximal penile numbness, which is usually transient and probably related to the division of the suspensory ligament (34). Overall, as for arterial revascularization procedures, initial enthusiasm for surgical treatment of veno-occlusive ED has been tempered by disappointing long-term results.

VACUUM ERECTION DEVICE

The need for a safe, reliable, reversible, noninvasive treatment for ED led to the development of the vacuum constriction device (VCD) in the 1980s. VCDs work by exerting a negative pressure on the penis resulting in increased corporeal blood flow and tumenescence. A constriction ring is then placed around the base of the penis to prolong the erection by obstructing drainage. Lederer (35) first patented the concept of a vacuum device used in conjunction with a compression ring in 1917. Credit for the popularization of the VCD, however, goes to Geddins Osbon who was granted permission by the US Food and Drug Administration (FDA) to market the device as the prescription device ErecAid (36). Although VCDs were initially viewed as a method to improve partial impotence or as an interim or alternative to first-line therapies, they have been widely recognized as a viable first-line treatment option since the early 1990s. Before the introduction of sildenafil, it was estimated that ~25% of the entire population of men with ED were using vacuum therapy for long-term management.

The literature reports successful erections in 84–95% of patients (37–39), with the overall satisfaction rate between 72% and 94% (40,41). The largest patient database is held by Osbon (ErecAid), who sent questionnaires to the 33,690 users in 1995. Ninety-nine percent reported good initial response and at 3 months, 77% were still using the ErecAid.

Complications of VCDs are few, but Peyronie's disease, skin necrosis, and petechia have been reported. Besides the up-front cost to purchase the VCDs, one of the disadvantages is the loss of spontaneity and the awkwardness of the device.

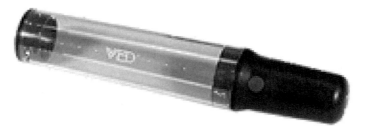

Figure 13.2 Vacuum constricting device.

Painful ejaculation has been reported in 10–15% of men due to compression of the urethra by the constriction device. VCDs are contraindicated in patients with bleeding disorders, but overall have a low incidence of side effects and are often effective in patients who have failed with other therapies. Gould reported that 71% of patients who failed with intracavernous injections obtained adequate rigidity with VCD (42) (Fig. 13.2).

INTRACAVERNOUS INJECTION THERAPY

Since the initial reports by Virag (43) and Brindley (44), intracorporeal self-injection of vasoactive agents has been widely used for the nonsurgical treatment of ED. The first reported self-injection program used a combination of papaverine and phentolamine and has proven to be a safe and satisfactory treatment for ED (45). These findings have since been validated by many subsequent large published series (46). Papaverine, phentolamine, and prostaglandin E1 (PGE1) are currently the most commonly used intracavernous agents for impotence therapy, typically combined as papaverine/phentolamine or as a combination of all three ("trimix"). Other agents such as moxisylyte chlorhydrate (Icavex) and vasoactive intestinal peptide (VIP) have also been shown to be effective.

Indications for self-injection therapy include mild to moderate arteriogenic and/or venogenic ED, psychogenic ED refractory to medical therapy, drug-induced ED, and failure of sildenafil therapy. General contraindications include a history of priapism, severe coagulopathy, unreliable or noncompliant patients, psychological instability, and poor manual dexterity.

Patients must receive appropriate training and education by medical personnel before beginning home injections. Adherence to correct technique can help reduce common side effects like hematomas, plaques, or fibrosis. Most importantly, after the first injection in the clinic, whether a full erection is produced or not, the patient should be educated about the risk of prolonged erection, an erection persisting greater than 4 h. The goal is to determine the lowest effective dose needed to produce an erection that is adequate for sexual intercourse that will be maintained for a reasonable time. This is best undertaken by dose escalation after taking into consideration the history, medication, and clinical findings to determine the initial dose.

All agents used for intracavernous self-injection therapy employ the same basic technique for administration. After the injection site is cleaned with alcohol, a 1 mL syringe and a 27–30 gauge needle are used to inject the penile corpora cavernosa at the 1 to 3 o'clock position or the 9 to 11 o'clock position to avoid the urethra ventrally and the neurovascular complex dorsally. The tip of the needle should be perpendicular to the skin to ensure proper, safe placement. Compression of the injection site for 5 min (10 min in men taking an anticoagulant drug) helps prevent hematomas. Visual or manual genital stimulation may confer a better result. Most patients cope well with the injection, although abdominal obesity, poor eyesight, and deficient manual dexterity can be obstacles to successful injection. In such patients, an auto-injector or partner may help.

Although the overall response rate is high, in long-term studies 38–80% of men cease self-injection therapy for various reasons not related to the efficacy of the therapy, including inconvenience, pain at the injection site, loss of partner, and the occurrence of side effects (47,48). Patient education regarding realistic results and complications as well as proper patient selection are important for ensuring the success of therapy.

Papaverine and Phentolamine

Papaverine, an alkaloid isolated from opium poppy, acts as a nonspecific phosphodiesterase inhibitor that increases cyclic AMP and cyclic GMP concentrations in penile erectile tissue for cavernous smooth muscle relaxation (49). Up to 80% of men with psychogenic and neurogenic ED have successful erections with papaverine, but only 36–50% of men with vasculogenic ED achieve this success. Papaverine for the treatment of ED is an off-label use and is unlicensed for intracavernosal injection in the USA.

Phentolamine, a nonselective alpha-adrenergic receptor antagonist, also causes smooth muscle relaxation with a half-life of only 30 min. When used alone, phentolamine does not produce rigid erections (50), but in combination with papaverine, success rates range from 63% to 87% (51,52). Most urologists prescribe a combination of 20–30 mg of papaverine and 0.5–1 mg of phentolamine, with the usual dose range from 0.1 mL to 1 mL.

Its low cost and easy storage makes papaverine appealing, but users need to be aware of the possible complications: priapism (35%), corporal fibrosis (33%), elevated serum aminotransferase concentrations, dizziness, pallor, cold sweats, and hypotension. The side effects of phentolamine include hypotension, reflex tachycardia, nasal congestion, gastrointestinal upset, and occasionally priapism.

Papaverine alone and papaverine–phentolamine mixture have formed the basis for self-injection programs for the management of ED since the mid

1980s. Mainly because of the risk of priapism and cavernosal fibrosis (46,52–55) there has been a move toward the use of PGE1.

Alprostadil

Three formulations of alprostadil are available for intracavernous injection: Prostin VR (Pharmacia & Upjohn); Caverject (Pharmacia & Upjohn), a lyophilized powder; and Edex (Schwarz Pharma), which contains alprostadil in complex with (alpha)-cyclodextrin. Alprostadil is the only intracavernous drug approved in the USA. Despite the diverse case mix presented to clinicians, numerous studies substantiate the efficacy of alprostadil. In a study by Stakl et al. (56), 70% of 550 patients reported a full erection lasting over 30 min, and all erections were adequate for vaginal penetration. Another large study by Porst (57) reported full erections in almost 73% of 10,353 patients with 70% patient satisfaction. In a variable-dose study of 683 men, 87–91% of patients reported satisfactory sexual performance (58). Satisfaction rates between 77% and 86% among partners were also reported (58,59). Overall, the efficacy of alprostadil is superior to that of papaverine and the combination of papaverine–phentolamine, resulting in erections in more than 70% of men (60–62).

In those with psychogenic, neurogenic, or unknown etiology of ED, the appropriate initial test dose of alprostadil is 2.5–5.0 μg, increasing in increments of 2.5 μg if necessary. In the elderly population with vascular disease or those with diabetes mellitus, it may be necessary to start with 10–20 μg. If this produces moderate tumescence only, then a combination of papaverine and PGE1 may be added. In a single-blind, dose-escalation study of 201 men, Linet and Ogrine (58) found the median effective dose to be 3.0, 4.0, and 5.0 μg in the psychogenic, neurogenic, and vasculogenic groups, respectively, to achieve 70% rigidity for greater than 10 min. Once confident in self-injection and alternating sites of injection, a maximum usage of one injection per 24 h and no more than three doses of alprostadil per week have been advised in the manufacturer's product information instructions.

The principal adverse effects from intracavernosal alprostadil are local: pain on injection (17–34%) (62–64), hematoma (1.5%), hemosiderin deposits (0.1%) (65), penile fibrosis, and Peyronie's plaque. Pain with injections is usually mild and rarely interferes with sexual intercourse. Nevertheless, painful erections are more prominent in men with partial nerve injury, such as those with diabetic neuropathy or those who have undergone radical pelvic surgery. Some patients find that the degree of discomfort after PGE1 injection inhibits their sexual enjoyment, leading to early discontinuation of treatment. The incidence of penile fibrosis arising from the use of intracavernosal injections is very difficult to quantify. Poor injection technique may account for local thickening of the tunica at the site of injection. Often, these nodules and areas of local fibrosis resolve. However, there is solid evidence showing corporeal fibrosis occurring at other sites away from the injection, and it can be extensive.

In a detailed study of patients receiving PGE1 for ED, Chew et al. (66) found that 57 of 245 patients (23.3%) developed penile fibrosis. The mean number of injections was 5.2 per month (range 1–16) for 29.7 months (range 2–86). This disturbingly high incidence of corporeal fibrosis had not been noted previously in the published literature. In a 15 year review of injection therapy involving 20,000 patients and 250,000 injections, Juenemann et al. (67) reported the incidence of fibrosis with papaverine to be 5% and only 2.5% with PGE1. The reason for this discrepancy is not obvious, but the findings of Chew et al. serve as a warning to those supervising self-injection programs not only to inform the patient of the possibility of penile fibrosis, but also to periodically check for its existence, which may be significantly higher than previously suspected.

Compared with papaverine and phentolamine, alprostadil is associated with a relatively low incidence of priapism (0.35–4%) and fibrosis (1–23%) (57,62,64,68). Another interesting side effect of alprostadil is spontaneous erections. In a recent study, a return of spontaneous erections increased throughout the study compared with baseline (37%) and was confirmed by interview for 46 of 54 (85%) men (69).

Systemic adverse outcomes have been reported but are uncommon for alprostadil. PGE1 is a vasodilator and systemic absorption could lead to hypotension, dizziness, or syncope. Other systemic side effects reported include abnormalities in liver function tests (70). PGE1 is present in human tissues (71). No significant rise in the levels of PGE1 was detected in the systemic circulation after intracavernosal injection, as it is metabolized by the lungs with a half-life of about 1 min (63).

Combinations of alprostadil with papaverine (72), ketanserin (73), or phentolamine (74) have proved superior to alprostadil alone. The most effective intracavernous therapy used in the USA is a three-drug mixture containing papaverine, phentolamine, and alprostadil (trimix). The usual dose of trimix solution ranges from 0.1 to 0.5 mL. The rate of response to this solution is as high as 90% (75). Although the trimix formulation has not been approved by the FDA, it is widely used in the USA.

Moxisylyte Chlorhydrate (Icavex)

Moxisylyte is a competitive noradrenaline antagonist, acting preferentially on postsynaptic alpha-1 adrenoceptors. It was introduced more than 30 years ago for the treatment of cerebrovascular disorders and has shown more recent efficacy in modulating urethral pressure (76). Renewed interest in this drug has been observed in recent years since the demonstration of the success of vasoactive drugs in ED treatment.

Intracavernous injections of moxisylyte at 10, 20, or 30 mg have induced erections adequate for intercourse in most patients. Recent studies have more often cited response rates ranging from 40% to 62%, which is significantly less effective compared with injectable agents such as papaverine and

PGE1 (77–82). At present, moxisylyte is mainly indicated in patients with super-sensitivity to injection of other agents and in those with significant pain or priapism following injection of PGE1 and papaverine.

Vasoactive Intestinal Polypeptide

VIP is a potent smooth-muscle relaxant originally isolated from the small intestine. Some evidence suggests that VIP is a neurotransmitter in the regulation of penile erections (83). Polak et al. (84) reported a decreased concentration of VIP in the penis of impotent men. Wagner and Gerstenberg (85) observed that intra-cavernosal injection of VIP in normal men produced tumescence but not rigidity.

When VIP is combined with phentolamine, the majority of men with mixed etiologies of ED appear to respond. Using 30 µg of VIP, and 0.5 to 2 mg of phen-tolamine with sexual stimulation, 52 men achieved a 100% success rate in attaining erection sufficient for intercourse (86). No episodes of priapism or corporeal fibrosis were reported. Dinsmore and Alderdice (87) reported that 67% of 70 men had erections sufficient for sexual intercourse. The combination of VIP and phentolamine thus appears to be a reasonable alternative to PGE1. Studies with longer follow-up suggest that it is safe, effective in a wide range of patients, and associated with less pain (88). Unfortunately, this combination is available in Europe, but not in the USA. Common side effects include transient facial flushing (53%), bruising (20%), pain at the injection site (11%), and truncal flushing (9%).

Despite the likely development of effective oral agents for ED and alternative methods of delivery of vasoactive agents via transdermal and urethral application, the use of intracorporeal agents will retain an important role in the management of ED. Some men alternate injection therapy with sildenafil or trans-urethral alprostadil, preferring injection when an erection of longer duration is desired. In refractory cases, combination therapy may prove to be very effective where monotherapy has failed, and some cases refractory to sildenafil respond to intracavernous injection. These findings imply that intracavernous injection remains an effective treatment option for ED (89).

MEDICATED URETHRAL SYSTEM FOR ERECTION

Demonstrating an efficacy of approximately 40–50% in early clinical trials, transurethral administration of PGE1 (alprostadil) was approved by the FDA in January 1997 for the treatment of ED. Alprostadil is a stable, synthetic form of PGE1, an endogenous unsaturated 20-carbon fatty-acid derivative of arachidonic acid. A small suppository of alprostadil is placed in the urethra and is absorbed through the urethral mucosa and corpus spongiousum. Within 10 min, a portion is transferred into the corpora cavernosa via small vascular communi-cations between the spongiosum and cavernosa (90). The maximal transfer occurs at 20–25 min, and the duration is ~1 h.

Initial trials of transurethral administration of alprostadil claim 50% success with fewer side effects than intracorporeal injection of alprostadil (91,92). There is, however, marked interpatient and intrapatient variability, and the clinical data reflect this with efficacy ranging from 13% to 66% (93). In two large, multicenter, double-blinded, placebo-controlled clinical trials conducted in the USA (92) and Europe (94), transurethral alprostadil was effective in 43% of men with ED from various organic causes. Guay et al. (95) have cited higher efficacy of transurethral administration of alprostadil (56%) than the initially published clinical trial and have recently reported clinical experiences with higher doses of alprostadil (500 μg in 49.2% and 1000 μg in 42.2%). Padma-Nathan et al. (92) found 65.9% of the men in clinic testing to have erections adequate for intercourse with MUSE and 64.9% of these responders achieved intercourse at least once during the 3 months that they treated themselves at home. On the other hand, Fulgham et al. (93) found that, independent of age and etiology, no more than 30% of patients (range 13–30%) at any given time using any dose achieved erections sufficient for intercourse during office testing. More than 80% of patients chose not to continue the use of MUSE at home.

Given the range of efficacy and side effects found in patients, patient selection is important. The use of intraurethral alprostadil administration ultimately depends on the patient's level of satisfaction with the quality of the erection. The first application, usually 500 μg, should be undertaken in the physician's office because of the potential complications of urethral bleeding, vasovagal reflex, hypotension, and priapism. Depending on the erectile response, the patient can be instructed to titrate the dose of alprostadil to effect (maximum of 1000 μg per dose).

The advantages of intraurethral therapy include local application, minimal systemic effects, and the rarity of drug interactions. Intraurethral administration of alprostadil can be efficacious in providing erections adequate for intercourse with lower risk of priapism than with intracavernosal injections (92). In addition to its use as monotherapy, transurethral alprostadil appears to augment other treatment modalities for ED. Benevides and Carson (96) found MUSE delivery of alprostadil to be efficacious in improving function of a penile prosthesis by engorging the glans penis. Combined therapy with sildenafil improved patient satisfaction and could be considered for those who had suboptimal response to monotherapy, refused it, or are nonsurgical candidates (97,98).

In comparison with intracavernosal injections, Porst (99) showed lower efficacy, higher side effects, and slower action with MUSE. Ghazi and Al Meligy (100) found that more patients preferred to continue intracavernosal injection than transurethral use. Even when comparing efficacy of alprostadil delivery via intracavernous injection vs. MUSE with an optional Actis ring, intracavernous injection therapy was more efficacious, better tolerated, and preferred by the patients and their partners (101). Although MUSE is less effective than intracavernosal PGE1, it is still an attractive option, suitable for a wide range of patients, especially those who are opposed to injections (102).

The major drawbacks of MUSE are moderate to severe penile pain, a low response rate, and inconsistent efficacy (99,103). Mild penile pain (10–29%) is the most common side effect (99,104). Intraurethral administraton of alprostadil may cause discomfort in pre-existing lower-limb varicosities, penile urethral discomfort, and possible vaginal discomfort for partners. This modality requires manual dexterity, good eyesight, and insertion after micturition. Men with significant venous leakage or spinal cord injury may be at greater risk of systemic hypotension. The use of an adjustable constriction device (Actis, Vivus, Mountain View, CA) placed at the base of the penis after the transurethral administration of alprostadil resulted in successful sexual intercourse in 69% (105) and may help reduce systemic effects of hypotension (106).

SILDENAFIL (VIAGRA)

Since its release in March 1998, sildenafil has become the drug of choice for most men with ED. Extensive media coverage has increased patient-driven demand for this product to levels unprecedented for any medication. There is no universally applicable treatment for ED, but, in appropriately selected patients, medical treatment can be very effective and is a well-established, first-line therapy for ED (17). It was hoped that sildenafil would prove to be close to the ideal pharmacologic treatment for ED—something that was effective, useful on demand, free of toxicity and side effects, easy to administer, and affordable (107). As expected, the introduction of sildenafil has also radically changed the medical approach to ED (108). No longer is an early referral to a specialist necessary. However, misconceptions about the efficacy, side effects, and safety persist, and the informed physician must still adjust expectations and communicate the availability of additional effective therapies.

Sildenafil is a selective inhibitor of phosphodiesterase type 5 which inactivates cyclic GMP and is found primarily within the corpora cavernosa (109). Sildenafil acts selectively in the penis to inhibit the breakdown of cyclic GMP, prolonging the duration and increasing the extent of cavernosal smooth-muscle relaxation, thereby enhancing and prolonging erection. Sildenafil requires sexual stimulation and at least, a partially intact penile nervous system to be efficacious since it has no direct relaxant effect on corporal smooth muscle but, rather, depends on the generation of nitric oxide and cyclic GMP. Sildenafil does not impact directly on libido, ejaculation, or orgasm (17,110).

Sildenafil is absorbed well during a fasting state, and the plasma concentrations are maximal within 30–120 min (mean 60 min). It is eliminated predominantly by hepatic metabolism, and the terminal half-life is about 4 h. The recommended starting dose is 50 mg taken 1 h before sexual activity, with the maximal recommended frequency of once per day. On the basis of effectiveness and side effects, the dose may be increased to a maximum of 100 mg or decreased to 25 mg.

In relatively healthy men (mean age 58 years), sildenafil was shown to treat ED successfully in a dose-dependent manner, with 69% of attempts being successful at the maximal dose of 100 mg given 60–90 min before intercourse (17). Overall, improvement in erectile response has been reported in 50–88% of patients (17,111). Sildenafil has been evaluated in 21 clinical trials of up to 6 months' duration in over 3000 men and in 10 open-label extension studies. Most of the men in these studies have organic or combined organic and psychogenic ED. The results were based mainly on the reports of the men, and sometimes the partners, and scores on the International Index of Erectile Function (IIEF). This index is a validated questionnaire with five domains: erectile function (six questions), orgasmic function (two questions), sexual desire (two questions), satisfaction with intercourse (three questions), and overall sexual satisfaction (two questions). In these studies, the number of erections and the quality of penile rigidity, orgasmic function, and overall sexual satisfaction were significantly higher with sildenafil than with placebo. In general, sildenafil works well for psychogenic and mild to moderate cases of organic ED. The efficacy is inferior but still substantial even in more severe organic ED.

Sildenafil has demonstrated effectiveness in men with ED associated with radical prostatectomy, radiation therapy, diabetes mellitus, certain neurologic disorders, and drug therapy selective serotonin reuptake inhibitors (112). Efficacy is about 50% in men with diabetes (113). There is limited efficacy after radical prostatectomy, and almost none if a non-nerve-sparing procedure has been done (114). Men with spinal cord injury experience improved erections, presumably through enhancement and prolongation of reflex erections (115).

Already considered by many to be the first-line therapy in most cases of ED, sildenafil certainly compares favorably to currently available ED therapy. Compared with other forms of ED treatment, sildenafil has been shown to be a cost-effective option to society based on the improved quality of life that can be attributed to this medication as well as the easier distribution through primary care physicians (116). Patients who already respond to intracavernous injection therapy can be switched over to oral sildenafil therapy with good satisfaction (up to 75%), tolerability, and efficacy (69–75%) (117,118). Moreover, though clinical data show sildenafil to be successful in 50–85% patients, that also implies that it is ineffective in 15–50% of patients with ED. Based on clinical experience with other pharmacotherapeutic agents for ED, combination and multi-agent therapy may prove more effective in men who do not respond to single-agent treatment. Sildenafil alone or sildenafil plus intracavernosal injection has been found to be effective salvage therapy for those not responding to intracavernosal injection. However, sildenafil in combination with intracavernosal injection is associated with a 33% incidence of adverse effects, including a 20% incidence of dizziness (119). Likewise, alprostadil injection therapy can be used effectively and safely in men who fail initial therapy with sildenafil. Interestingly, up to 33% of intracavernous injection therapy users who responded to sildenafil chose to return to injection therapy (117). Thus, while sildenafil should be considered as first-line treatment, men with ED should be aware of all the treatment options available.

Overall, sildenafil appears to be well tolerated and safe for the majority of patients. Clinical safety has been evaluated in more than 3700 patients with 1631 patient-years of exposure to sildenafil. Most adverse events were mild to moderate and self-limited in duration (120). Among men taking 25 to 100 mg of sildenafil, 16% reported headache, 10% flushing, 7% dyspepsia, 4% nasal congestion, and 3% abnormal vision. These rates were twice as high among men taking 100 mg of sildenafil than among those who were on lower doses. The visual effect, described as a mild and transient blue color tinge or increased sensitivity to light, is related to the nonspecific inhibition of phosphodiesterase type 6 in the retina. The presence of retinitis pigmentosa is another concern, since some cases are thought to be due to a phosphodiesterase disorder. No chronic visual impairment has been reported to date, and the incidence of visual side effects is similar in diabetic and nondiabetic men (121). Nevertheless, because of the short duration of the clinical trials and the difficulty in detecting subtle retinal changes, the long-term safety of sildenafil treatment is unknown. In men with retinal diseases, an ophthalmologic consultation may be warranted before sildenafil treatment is initiated.

Adverse events (nasal congestion, headache, and flushing) were mild and transient in the majority of men. However, from late March to mid-November 1998, 130 deaths associated with sildenafil therapy were reported to the US FDA. During the same period, more than six million outpatient prescriptions of sildenafil were dispensed (about 50 million tablets) to more than three million men. It is difficult to gauge the relevance of sildenafil for many of the reported deaths given the limited amount of clinical data available, but the number of significant adverse events seems small given the large number of men who have taken the drug. Various anecdotal cardiac and vascular events have been reported, including myocardial infarction, arrhythmia, congestive heart failure, cerebrovascular accidents, and transient ischemic attacks. The reported rate of serious cardiovascular events (angina and coronary artery disorder) from March to November 1998 was 4.1 per 100 man-years of treatment among those taking sildenafil and 5.7 per 100 man-years for those taking placebo. The rates of myocardial infarction were 1.7 and 1.4 per 100 man-years for the sildenafil and placebo groups, respectively (120). Other reviews of clinical trials show that sildenafil is not associated with an increase in serious cardiovascular adverse events, myocardial infarction, or death compared to placebo (122).

In response to the concern of physicians, the American College of Cardiology and the American Heart Association have published guidelines for sildenafil therapy and have recommended that sildenafil use be treated with caution in men with active coronary disease who are not taking nitrates, men with heart failure and borderline low blood pressure or volume status, men on complicated multi-drug antihypertensive regimens, and men taking drugs that prolong the half-life of sildenafil (erythromycin, cimetidine, and ketoconazole) (17,123). Concomitant nitrate use can cause profound hypotension, and nitrate use remains the single definite contraindication to sildenafil. Given that most of the men who died had underlying cardiovascular disease, cardiovascular status should be carefully assessed before treatment.

OTHER ORAL AGENTS

Since the debut of sildenafil in 1998, other oral agents for ED have faded into the background. For the sake of completeness, these will be discussed as they are still available for use.

Herbal Therapy

In traditional Asian culture, centuries of clinical observation have led to the popular belief that Korean red ginseng is a valuable stimulant for health and sexual powers. The active ingredient of this ancient, herbal drug remains elusive, but research is focused on saponin, an extract. Ginseng's mechanism of action is believed to be a "combination of vasodilation, anti-depression, anxiolytic (anti-stress), and microvascular flow improvement" (124). The most plausible explanation is the antistress effect of ginseng, which brings improvement in androgen production and sexual function. In 1995, Choi reported a randomized, unblinded study comparing three groups for treatment of ED: Korean red ginseng, placebo, and trazadone. A total of 90 patients (30 patients in each group) were followed for 3 months. Therapeutic efficacy was evaluated by monthly interviews with the patient and partner. The overall therapeutic efficacy was 60% for ginseng, 30% for placebo, and 30% for trazadone. No complete response was noted, but ginseng was found to be significantly better than trazadone and placebo in treating ED. No complications were reported.

Trazadone

Another historic drug that warrants mention is trazadone, a serotonin antagonist and reuptake inhibitor. Anecdotal reports of improved sexual function in patients treated with trazadone for depression appeared in the psychiatric literature in 1985 (125). Trazadone is used primarily as a sedative and antidepressant, but was found to cause priapism in rare cases (1/10,000 users). The mechanism of action for erectile response is unknown, but it is believed to stimulate 5HT1c receptor, known for its libido-improving properties (126).

Meinhardt et al. (127) performed a double-blind, placebo-controlled, multi-center trial in 1997, and found no significant difference in the subjective results of 58 patients between placebo and trazadone. In 1999, Costabile and Spevale (125) restated that trazadone is no more effective than placebo in improving sexual dysfunction in his double-blind, placebo-controlled trial of 48 men. He postulated that with treatment of depression, improved erectile dysfunction is expected.

No serious adverse reactions with trazadone were reported, but the main side effects were nausea and drowsiness. Synergism with yohimbine has been suggested, but its beneficial effects have not been substantiated in a prospective, placebo-controlled, double-blinded trial.

Yohimbine

Yohimbine, an indole alkaloid from the bark of the Central African yohimbine tree, is an oral agent that had widespread used before the advent of sildenafil. It is a member of the adrenergic-receptor antagonist family, and produces a rise in central nervous system sympathetic drive by increasing noradrenaline release and by increasing the firing rate of cells located in noradrenergic nuclei (128). It presumably stimulates the brain center associated with libido and penile erections.

Ernst reviewed and meta-analyzed all randomized, placebo-controlled trials of yohimbine monotherapy. Seven trials that met the inclusion criteria demonstrated individually that yohimbine is superior to placebo. At present, it is not clear which type of ED responds best to yohimbine, but across all studies, responders vary from 34% to 73% (128). As with all meta-analyses, selection bias is an important consideration that may distort the overall results. The American Urologic Association (AUA) guidelines on treatment of organic ED point out the noticeable placebo effect, but the authors respond with the positive results of trials published after 1997 that were not included in the AUA evaluation. Unlike the data collected by the AUA strictly evaluating organic ED, the data of this meta-analysis describe less well-defined etiologies of ED and cannot be compared to the AUA results. Kunelius et al. (129) examined 29 patients with mixed-type ED in a prospective, randomized, controlled double-blind crossover study. No statistical difference in positive results was seen between placebo (48%) and high-dose yohimbine (44%). In 1998, Teloken et al. (130) evaluated men with organic ED treated with placebo and 100 mg yohimbine hydrochloride. No statistical difference was found in the 22 patients, mean age 58 years. Side effects are a result of noradrenergic activity and include anxiety, nausea, palpitations, fine tremors, and elevation of diastolic blood pressure (126).

Delaquamine and Phentolamine (Vasomax)

Other members of the adrenergic-receptor antagonist family include delaquamine and phentolamine. Delaquamine, a newer selective alpha-2 adrenoreceptor antagonist, is 100× more selective than yohimbine. Clinical studies have revealed some resumption of erectile function (131), but they are unable to prove efficacy over placebo (126).

Phentolamine, a nonselective alpha-blocker, has antiserotonin action and a direct nonspecific relaxant effect on blood vessels to facilitate erections (126). In an open-label trial, Zorgniotti (132) reports a 42% response rate in patients with mild ED with 50 mg of phentolamine HCl compared to 9% with 10 mg of phenoxybenzamine. A second single-blinded trial was performed in 68 new patients at a different time. There was a 32% success rate with 20 mg of phentolamine mesylate buccal tablet compared to 13% with the lactose placebo. Both oral and buccal phentolamine appear safe for ED, but further investigation of this drug is warranted. Side effects include stuffy nose (6%), faintness and/or dizziness (2%), and vomiting (<0.01%). Becker et al. (133) performed a prospective, double-blind, and placebo-controlled trial with oral phentolamine (20, 40, and 60 mg) and placebo. Out of 40 patients with less than a 3 year history of erectile dysfunction, full erections were achieved by 2 of 10 with placebo, 3 of 10 with 20 mg, 5 of 10 with 40 mg, and 4 of 10 with 60 mg phentolamine. The only side effect reported was a stuffy nose after 60 mg in one patient. Oral phentolamine is not FDA approved. Further clinical trials have been suspended due to liver toxicity found in animal models (134).

L-Arginine

In an approach to targeting ED peripherally, L-arginine, the precursor to nitric oxide (NO), has been used in experimental trials. NO, found in the endothelium of the penile cavernous space, is involved in the neurotransmission process that leads to smooth-muscle relaxation in the corpus cavernosum. This, in turn, increases the blood flow in the penile arteries and initiates penile erections. Since NO is derived from L-arginine, it has been suggested that supplementing this semi-amino acid substrate in impotent men may improve erectile function. Since the action of nitric oxide synthase (NOS) is the rate limiting step in this conversion, increased concentrations of L-arginine may not facilitate erections in humans. In the rat model, correction of age-associated ED was demonstrated with long-term administration of high-dose L-arginine, as measured by electrical field stimulation of the cavernosal nerve (135). The only study reported in human literature is a placebo-controlled, 2 week trial of large doses (2800 mg/day) of L-arginine (136). Fifteen men completed the treatment of 2 weeks of daily placebo and another 2 weeks of daily L-arginine. Six of 15 (40%) reported improved function with L-arginine compared to 0 of 15 with placebo. Further investigation is warranted to elicit if there is a deficit in NO or L-arginine in the responders.

Apomorphine (Uprima)

Apomorphine, a direct central D2 receptor agonist, is the first drug to restore erectile function through a central mechanism. A positive effect on sexual arousal was demonstrated in a rat model (137). Erection induced by the addition of apomorphine is natural in that it mimics the pattern of the unaided erection under study conditions. It is proposed to work centrally to enhance proerectile signaling through decreased inhibitory signals and augmenting of the normal pathways. Phase III trials began 4 years ago. Doses of apomorphine SL have peak serum levels that are several times lower (less than 1.5 ng/dL) than those required for direct vascular effects (126). Therefore, there is no basis to expect systemic vasodilation from apomorphine SL or interaction with cardiovascular medications, like nitrates. There are no reports of death, myocardial infarctions, cerebrovascular accident, or priapisms thus far. However, persistent yawning, nausea, vomiting, hypotension, and syncope have been cited (126).

Heaton (138) summarized an update on the first three phase III parallel arm crossover double-blind studies on apomorphine SL. Eight hundred fifty-four patients were given a total of 8263 tablets of apomorphine SL in 2 and 4 mg doses. Men between 18 and 70 years of age consented with their partner to attempt intercourse approximately twice a week for the duration of their participation. The majority (74.1%) had moderate and severe ED, 31% had hypertension, 16% had documented coronary artery disease, 16% had dyslipidemia, and 16% had diabetes. Erections occurred in 54.4% of attempts at 4 mg (vs. 33.8% with placebo), and 50.6% of attempts at intercourse were successful. The most common side effect was nausea, and 2.1% of patients on 2 mg experienced nausea at least once. This increased to 20.4% in patients on 4 mg of apomorphine SL. Nevertheless, nausea was found to have no impact on efficacy or trial dropout rate.

Cialis and Vardenafil

The direction of future oral agents is focused on cialis and vardenafil, both type 5 phosphodiesterase inhibitors. Like sildenafil, both agents work by prolonging the activity of cGMP, promoting cavernous smooth-muscle relaxation and enhancing erectile function. In a recent press release at the AUA meeting in June 2001 (139), Bayer reported positive results from a recent phase II, placebo-controlled double-blinded study involving 601 men. All domains of the IIEF were significantly improved over the 12 week study. By 4 weeks, vardenafil significantly improved all aspects of ED at all doses. The most common side effects include headaches, flushing, and nasal congestion. Bayer plans to submit a new drug application to the US FDA in the third quarter of 2001. In another press release, Lilly ICOS has submitted an application to the US FDA for cialis. At the 96th annual AUA meeting, they reported a prompt response and extended period of responsiveness for cialis, 20 mg. Compared to sildenafil, cialis has a shorter onset of action (16 min) and a much longer duration, up to 24 h. Commonly reported adverse effects include headache, back pain, and dyspepsia (140).

GENE THERAPY

The ultimate goal of medical therapy for ED is to correct the etiology of ED rather than supplement or support what remains and to achieve long-term erections naturally without pretreatment prior to sexual intercourse. A truly novel approach is to correct the fundamental biologic defect leading to ED. For instance, if NO production in the cavernosal endothelium was reduced or impaired, smooth muscle cannot relax and ED results. In turn, any pharmacologic supplementation of NO would correct the deficit, restoring smooth-muscle relaxation and erectile function. Instead of temporarily supplementing NO function with agents that would either supply NO precursors (L-arginine) or enhance the cGMP pathway (sildenafil), the novel biologic approach is to focus more attention toward gene transfer of cDNA to the target organ, in the hope of sustaining expression of the corresponding mRNA and maintaining physiological control of protein activity (135). This concept is gaining acceptance for possible treatment of inborn metabolic errors of metabolism and cancer using gene transfer with vectors such as liposomes or adenovirus. Cystic fibrosis, adenosine deaminase deficiency, and familial hypercholesterolemia are some of the diseases for which gene therapy has been successful.

An obvious candidate for gene therapy in ED is NOS cDNA (135). Recent studies have shown that tissue-specific NOS isoforms are expressed both in the rat and in the human penis. cDNA for both iNOS and nNOS have been cloned. Recent discovery of a penile nNOS variant, PnNOS, shows promise for gene therapy. It differs from the cerebellar nNOS in the presence of the 34-amino acid stretch that is likely to confer some unique regulatory function related to the role of NO in smooth-muscle relaxation. PnNOS is expressed as the dominant form of nNOS in the prostate and urethra, and is mixed with cerebellar nNOS in the bladder. This suggests that it is the main enzyme in the NO cascade that controls the tone in the lower urinary tract. With the feasibility of delivering biologically active modulators to the penis and manipulating penile NOS expression, the aging-associated ED may be corrected. A single injection of a construct of the RPiNOS coding region under the control of a strong promotor in a liposomal preparation, delivered to the corpora, achieved positive results lasting 10–14 days (135). The accessibility of the corpora cavernosa for direct drug delivery and the patient's acceptance of this route provide a unique advantage for studies of gene therapy of the penis compared to other organs.

CONCLUSIONS

It is difficult to believe that two decades ago, ED was considered a psychogenic disease with no effective therapy. Much has evolved in the science of ED, beginning with the establishment as an organic disorder. Since then, various approaches to therapy, maximally to minimally invasive, have brought more insight and understanding of ED. With the influence of mass media in exposing previously private subjects, the public's pursuit of improved quality of life has spurred the demand for additional minimally invasive therapies. Currently, clinical trials for more specific, effective oral therapies are under way. ED is a medically treatable disease that has wide-reaching consequence in a man's quality of life. Management of ED will be based on the patient's preference, cost, and comfort. The key to finding the most appropriate management will be eliciting the patient's and partner's preference and understanding their expectations.

REFERENCES

1. Lespinasse V. Impotency: its treatment by transplantation of the testicle. Surg Clin Chicago 1918; 2:281–288.
2. Voronoff S. Rejuvenation by Grafting. London: George Allen and Unwin, 1925.
3. Lower W. The exocrine and endocrine functions of the testis. J Urol 1934; 31:391–396.
4. Stekel W. Impotence in the Male. New York: Liveright, 1927.
5. Huhner M. Masterbation and impotence from a urological standpoint. J Urol 1936; 36:770–784.
6. Melman A, Gingell JC. The epidemiology and pathophysiology of erectile dysfunction. J Urol 1999; 161:5–11.
7. Furlow W. Prevalence of impotence in the United States. Med Aspects Hum Sex 1985; 19:13–17.
8. Feldman H, Goldstein I, Hatzichristou D, Krane R, McKinlay J. Impotence and its medical and psychosocial correlates: results of the Massachusetts male aging study. J Urol 1994; 151:54–61.
9. Laumann EO, Paik AM, Rosen RC. Sexual dysfunction in the United States: prevalence and predictors. J Am Med Assoc 1999; 281:537–544.
10. Wabrek A, Burchell R. Male sexual dysfunction associated with coronary heart disease. Arch Sex Behav 1980; 9:69–75.
11. Gundle M, Reeves B, Tate S, Raft D, McLaurin L. Psychological outcome after aortocoronary artery surgery. Am J Psychiatry 1980; 137:1591–1594.
12. Fairbairn C, McCulloch D, Wu F. The effects of diabetes on male erectile dysfunction. Baillieres Clin Endocrinol Metab 1982; 11:749–784.
13. Hakim L. Diabetic sexual dysfunction. Endocrinol Metab Clin North Am 1996; 25:379–400.
14. Rosen M, Greenfield A, Walker T, Grant P, Dubrow J, Bettmann M, Fried L, Goldstein I. Cigarette smoking: an independent risk factor for atherosclerosis in the hypogastric-cavernous arterial bed of men with arteriogenic impotence. J Urol 1991; 146:759–763.
15. Buffum J. Pharmacosexology: the effects of drugs on sexual function—a review. J Psychoactive Drugs 1982; 14:5–44.
16. Benet A, Melman A. The epidemiology of erectile dysfunction. Urol Clin North Am 1995; 22:699–709.
17. Goldstein I, Lue T, Padma-Nathan H, Rosen R, Steer W, Wicker P. Oral sildenafil in the treatment of erectile dysfunction. N Engl J Med 1998; 338:1397–1404.
18. Bergman R, Howard A, Barnes R. Plastic reconstruction of the penis. J Am Med Assoc 1948; 59:1174–1180.
19. Loeffler R, Savegh E, Lash H. The artificial os penis. Plast Reconstr Surg 1964; 34:71–74.
20. Mulcahy J. Unitary inflatable, mechanical and malleable penile implants. In: Carson C, Kirby R, Goldstein I, eds. Textbook of Erectile Dysfunction. Oxford: ISIS Medical Media, 1999:413–421.

21. Carson C. Inflatable penile prosthesis. In: Carson C, Kirby R, Goldstein I, eds. Textbook of Erectile Dysfunction. Oxford: ISIS Medical Media, 1999:423–433.
22. Carson C, Mulcahy J, Govier F. Efficacy, safety and patient satisfaction outcomes of the AMS 700CX inflatable penile prosthesis: results of a long-term multicenter study. AMS 700CX Study Group. J Urol 2000; 164:376–380.
23. Chiang H. 10 years of experience with penile prosthesis implantation in Taiwanese patient. J Urol 2000; 163:476–480.
24. Carson C. Complications of penile prostheses and complex implantations. In: Carson C, Kirby R, Goldstein I, eds. Textbook of Erectile Dysfunction. Oxford: ISIS Medical Media. 1999:435–450.
25. Garber B. Inflatable penile prosthesis: results of 150 cases. Br J Urol 1996; 78:933–935.
26. Michal V, Kramar R, Pospichal J, Hejhal L. Direct arterial anastomosis to the cavernous body in the treatment of erectile impotence. Czech Rozhledy Chir 1973; 52:587–590.
27. Anafarta K, Aydos K, Yaman O. Is deep dorsal vein arterialization an alternative surgical approach to treat venogenic impotence? Urol Int 1997; 59:109–112.
28. Hauri D. Penile revascularization surgery in erectile dysfunction. Andrologia 1999; 31S:65–76.
29. Goldstein I. Arterial revascularization procedures. Semin Urol 1986; 4:252–258.
30. Zumbe J, Scheidhauer K, Kieslich F, Heidenreich A, Klotz T, Vorreuther R, Engelman U. Nuclear medical assessment of penile hemodynamics following revascularization surgery. Urol Int 1997; 58:39–42.
31. Wespes E, Schulman C. Venous leakage: surgical treatment of a curable cause of impotence. J Urol 1985; 133:796–798.
32. Lue T. Surgery for crural venous leakage. Urology 1999; 54:739–741.
33. Schulthesis D, Truss M, Becker A, Steif C, Jonas U. Long-term results following dorsal penile vein ligation in 126 patients with veno-occlusive dysfunction. Int J Impot Res 1997; 9:205–209.
34. Lue T. Penile venous surgery. Urol Clin North Am 1989; 16:607–611.
35. Lederer O. Specification of letter patent. United States Patent Office #1, 225, 341, May 8, 1917.
36. Witherington R. The Osbon ErecAid system in the management of erectile impotence. J Urol 1985; 133:190A.
37. Witherington R. Vacuum constriction device for management of erectile dysfunction. J Urol 1989; 141:320–322.
38. Turner L, Althof S, Levine S, Bodner D, Kursh E, Resnick M. External vacuum devices in the treatment of erectile dysfunction: a one year study of sexual and psychological impact. J Sex Marital Ther 1991; 17:81–93.
39. Cookson M, Nadig P. Long term results with vacuum constriction device. J Urol 1993; 149:290–294.
40. Moul J, McLeod D. Negative pressure devices in the explanterectile dysfunction prosthesis population. J Urol 1989; 142:729–731.
41. Baltaci S, Aydos K, Kosar A, Anafarta K. Treating erectile dysfunction with a vacuum tumescence device: a retrospective analysis of acceptance and satisfaction. Br J Urol 1995; 76:757–760.
42. Oakley N, Allen P, Moore T. Vacuum devices for erectile impotence. In: Carson C, Kirby R, Goldstein I, eds. Textbook of Erectile Dysfunction. Oxford: ISIS Medical Media, 1999;371–381.

43. Virag R. Intracavernous injection of papaverine for erectile failure. Lancet 1982; 11:938–942.
44. Brindley G. Cavernosal alpha blockage: a new technique for investigating and treating erectile impotence. Br J Psychiatry 1983; 143:332–337.
45. Zorgniotti A, Lefleur R. Autoinjection of the corpus cavernosum with a vasoactive drug combination for vasculogenic impotence. J Urol 1985; 133:39–41.
46. Lakin M, Montague D, Mendendorp S, Tesar L, Schover L. Intracavernous injection therapy: analysis of results and complications. J Urol 1990; 143:1138–1141.
47. Weiss J, Badlani G, Ravalli R, Brettschneider N. Reasons for high drop-out rate with self-injection therapy for impotence. Int J Impot Res 1994; 6:171–174.
48. Gupta R, Krishen J, Barrow RI, Eid J. Predictors of success and risk factors for attrition in the use of intracavernous injection. J Urol 1997; 157:1681–1686.
49. Jeremy J, Ballard S, Naylor A, Miller M, Angelini G. Effects of sildenafil, a type-5-cGMP phosphodiesterase inhibitor, and papaverine on cyclic GMP and cyclic AMP levels in the rabbit corpus cavernosum in vitro. Br J Urol 1997; 79:958–963.
50. Steif C, Wetterauer U. Erectile responses to intracavernous papaverine and phentolamine: comparison of single and combined delivery. J Urol 1988; 140:1415–1416.
51. Fallon B. Intracavernous injection therapy for male erectile dysfunction. Urol Clin North Am 1995; 22:833–845.
52. Juenemann K, Alken P. Pharmacotherapy of erectile dysfunction: a review. Int J Impot Res 1989; 1:71–93.
53. Levine S, Althol S, Turner L, Risen C, Bodner D, Kursh E, Resnick M. Side effects of self-administration of intracavernous papaverine and phentolamine for the treatment of impotence. J Urol 1989; 141:54–57.
54. Hu K-N, Burks C, Christy WC. Fibrosis of tunica albuginea: complication of long-term intracavernous pharmacological self-injection. J Urol 1987; 138:404–405.
55. Abozeid M, Junemann K, Luo J, Lue T, Yen T, Tanagho E. Chronic papaverine treatment: the effect of repeated injections on the simian erectile response and penile tissue. J Urol 1987; 138:1263–1266.
56. Stackl W, Hanson R, Marberger M. The use of prostaglandin E1 for the diagnosis and treatment of erectile dysfunction. World J Urol 1990; 8:84–86.
57. Porst H. The rational for prostaglandin E1 in erectile failure: a survey of worldwide experience. J Urol 1996; 155:802–815.
58. Linet O, Ogrine F. Efficacy and safety of intracavernosal alprostadil in men with erectile dysfunction. New Engl J Med 1996; 334:873–877.
59. Porst H, van Ahlen H, Block T, Halbig W, Hautmann R, Lochner-Ernst D, Rudnick J, Staehler G, Weber H, Weidner W. Intracavernous self-injection of prostaglandin E1 in the therapy of erectile dysfunction. Vasa Suppl 1989; 28:50–56.
60. Stackl W, Hanson R, Marberger M. Intracavernous injection of prostaglandin E1 in impotent men. J Urol 1988; 140:66–68.
61. Lee L, Stevenson R, Szasz G. Prostaglandin E1 versus phentolamine/papaverine for the treatment of erectile impotence: a double-blind comparison. J Urol 1989; 141:549–550.
62. Linet O, Neff L. Intracavernous prostaglandin E1 in erectile dysfunction. Clin Invest 1994; 72:139–149.
63. Pryor J. Caverject and erectile dysfunction. J Sex Health 1994; S4–S5.

64. Chew K, Stuckey B, Earle C, Dhaliwal S, Keogh E. Penile fibrosis in intracavernosal prostaglandin E1 injection therapy for erectile dysfunction. Int J Impot Res 1997; 9:225–229.

65. Krane R, Goldstein I, Saenz de Tejada I. Impotence. New Engl J Med 1989; 321:1648–1659.

66. Chew K, Earle C, Stuckley B, Keogh E. Penile fibrosis in intracavernosal PGE1 injection therapy for erectile dysfunction. Int J Impot Res 1996; 8:143–146.

67. Juenemann K, Manning M, Krautschick A, Alken P. 15 years of injection therapy in erectile dysfunction—a review. Int J Impot Res 1996; 8:14–18.

68. Canale D, Giorgi P, Lencioni R, Morelli G, Gasperi M, Macchia E. Long-term intracavernous self-injection with prostaglandin E1 for the treatment of erectile dysfunction. Int J Androl 1996; 19:28–32.

69. Brock G, Tu L, Linet O. Return of spontaneous erection during long-term intracavernosal alprostadil (Caverject) treatment. Urology 2001; 57:536–541.

70. Anderson K, Holmquist F, Wagner G. Pharmacology of drugs used for treatment of erectile dysfunction and priapism. Int J Impot Res 1991; 6:155–172.

71. Templeton A, Cooper T, Kelly R. Prostaglandin concentrations in the semen of fertile men. J Reprod Fertil 1978; 58:147–150.

72. Zaher T. Papaverine plus prostaglandin E1 versus prostaglandin E1 alone for intracorporeal injection therapy. Int Urol Nephrol 1998; 30:193–196.

73. Mirone V, Imbimbo C, Fabrizio F, Longo N, Palmieri A. Ketanserin plus prostaglandin E1 (PGE-1) as intracavernosal therapy for patients with erectile dysfunction unresponsive to PGE-1 alone. Br J Urol 1996; 77:736–739.

74. Meinhardt W, de la Fuente R, Lycklama a Nijeholt A, Vermeij P, Zwartendijk J. Prostaglandin E1 with phentolamine for the treatment of erectile dysfunction. Int J Impot Res 1996; 8:5–7.

75. Bennett A, Carpenter A, Barada J. An improved vasoactive drug combination for a pharmacological erection program. J Urol 1991; 146:1564–1565.

76. Marquer C, Bressolle F. Moxisylyte: a review of its pharmacodynamic and pharmacokinetic properties, and its therapeutic use in impotence. Fundam Clin Pharmacol 1998; 12:377–387.

77. Navratil H, Costa P, Louis J, Andro M, Saur P. Effectiveness of and tolerance to intracavernous injection of moxisylyte in patients with erectile dysfunction: effect/dose relationship versus placebo. Prog Urol 1995; 5:690–696.

78. Buvat J, Costa P, Morlier D, Lecocq B, Stegmann B, Albrecht D. Double-blind multicenter study comparing alprostadil alpha-cyclodextrin with moxisylyte chlorhydrate in patients with chronic erectile dysfunction. J Urol 1998; 159:116–119.

79. Buvat J, Costa P, Morlier D, Lecocq B, Stegmann B, Albrecht D. Erectile response to intracavernosal injection of alprostadil compared with moxisylyte chlorhydrate in chronic erectile dysfunction: a double-blind, multi-centre study in 156 patients. Int J Impot Res 1996; 8:114–117.

80. Buvat J, Lemaire A, Herbaut-Buvat M. Intracavernous pharmacotherapy: comparison of moxisylyte and prostaglandin E1. Int J Impot Res 1996; 8:41–46.

81. Hermabessiere J, Costa P, Andro M. Efficacy and tolerance of intracavernous injection of moxisylyte in patients with erectile dysfunction: double-blind placebo-controlled study. Prog Urol 1995; 5:985–991.

82. Buvat J, Buvat-Herbaut M, Lemaire A, Marcolin G. Treatment of impotence with intracavernous auto-injections: moxisylyte diminishes the risks compared to papaverine. Contracept Fertil Sex 1993; 21:173–176.
83. Ottesen B, Wagner G, Virag R, Fahrenkrug J. Penile erection: possible role for vasoactive intestinal polypeptide as a neurotransmitter. Br Med J 1984; 288:9–12.
84. Polak J, Gu J, Mina S, Bloom S. VIPergic nerves in the penis. Lancet 1981; 2:217–220.
85. Wagner G, Gerstenberg T. Intracavernosal injection of vasoactive intestinal polypeptide (VIP) does not induce erection in man per se. World J Urol 1987; 5:171–174.
86. Gerstenberg T, Metz P, Ottensen B, Fahrenkrug J. Intracavernous self-injection with vasoactive intestinal polypeptide and phentolamine in the management of erectile failure. J Urol 1992; 147:1277–1279.
87. Dinsmore W, Alderdice D. Vasoactive intestinal polypeptide and phentolamine mesylate administered by autoinjector in the treatment of patients with erectile dysfunction resistant to other intracavernosal agents. Br J Urol 1998; 81:437–440.
88. Gerstenberg T. Long term use of vasopotin in the treatment of erectile dysfunction. Int J Impot Res 1995; 7:5–8.
89. McMahon C, Samali R, Johnson H. Efficacy, safety, and patient acceptance of sildenafil citrate as treatment for erectile dysfunction. J Urol 2000; 164:1192–1196.
90. Vardi Y, Saenz de Tejada I. Functional and radiologic evidence of vascular communication between the spongiosal and cavernous compartments of the penis. Urology 1997; 49:749–752.
91. Hellstrom W, Bennett A, Gesundheit N, Kaiser F, Lue T, Padma-Nathan H, Peterson C, Tam P, Todd L, Varady J, Place V. A double-blind, placebo controlled evaluation of the erectile response to transurethral alprostadil. Urology 1996; 48:851–856.
92. Padma-Nathan H, Hellstrom W, Kaiser F, Labasky R, Lue T, Nolton W, Norwood P, Peterson C, Shabsigh R, Tam P, Place V, Gesundheit N, Cowley C, Nem K, Spivack A, Stephens D, Todd L. For the Medicated Urethral System for Erection (MUSE) Study Group: treatment of men with erectile dysfunction with transurethral alprostadil. N Engl J Med 1997; 336:1–7.
93. Fulgham P, Cochran J, Denman J, Feagins B, Gross M, Kadesky K, Kadesky M, Clark A, Roehrborn C. Disappointing initial results with transurethral alprostadil for erectile dysfunction in a urology practice setting. J Urol 1998; 160:2041–2046.
94. Williams G, Abbou C, Amar E, Desvaux P, Flam T, Lycklama a Nijeholt G, Lynch S, Morgan R, Muller S, Porst H, Pryor J, Ryan P, Witzsch U, Hall M, Place V, Spivack A, Gesundheit N. Efficacy and safety of transurethral alprostadil therapy in men with erectile dysfunction. Br J Urol 1998; 81:889–894.
95. Guay A, Perez J, Velasquez E, Newton R, Jacobson J. Clinical experience with intraurethral alprostadil (MUSE) in the treatment of men with erectile dysfunction. A retrospective study. Medicated urethral system for erection. Eur Urol 2000; 38:671–676.
96. Benevides M, Carson C. Intraurethral application of alprostadil in patients with failed inflatable penile prosthesis. J Urol 2000; 163:785–787.
97. Mydlo J, Volpe M, MacChia R. Results from different patient populations using combined therapy with alprostadil and sildenafil: predictors of satisfaction. BJU Int 2000; 86:469–473.

98. Mydlo J, Volpe M, MacChia R. Initial results utilizing combination therapy for patients with a suboptimal response to either alprostadil or sildenafil monotherapy. Eur Urol 2000; 38:30–34.

99. Porst H. Transurethral alprostadil with MUSETM (medicated urethral system for erection) vs intracavernous alprostadil—a comparative study in 103 patients with erectile dysfunction. Int J Impot Res 1997; 9:187–192.

100. Ghazi S, Al Meligy A. Transurethral alprostadil and the prostaglandin E1 intracorporal injection in treatment of erectile dysfunction: a comparative study. Int J Impot Res 1998; 10:S13.

101. Shabsigh R, Padma-Nathan H, Gittleman M, McMurray J, Kaufman J, Goldstein I. Intracavernous alprostadil alfadex is more efficacious, better tolerated, and preferred over intraurethral alprostadil plus optional actis: a comparative, randomized, crossover, multicenter study. Urology 2000; 55:109–113.

102. Shokeir A, Alserafi M, Mutabagani H. Intracavernosal versus intraurethral alprostadil: a prospective, randomized study. BJU Int 1999; 83:812–815.

103. Werthman P, Rajfer J. MUSE therapy: preliminary clinical observations. Urology 1997; 50:809–811.

104. Hellstrom W, Peterson C, Tam P. One-year study of transurethral alprostadil for erectile dysfunction: efficacy, safety, and satisfaction (for the MUSE Study Group). Int J Impot Res 1998; 10:S49.

105. Lewis R. Combined use of transurethral alprostadil and an adjustable penile constriction band in men with erectile dysfunction: results from a multicenter trial. J Urol 1998; 159:237A.

106. Bodner D, Haas C, Krueger B, Seftel A. Intraurethral alprostadil for treatment of erectile dysfunction in patients with spinal cord injury. Urology 1999; 53:199–202.

107. Morales A, Heaton J, Johnston B, Adams M. Oral and topical treatment of erectile dysfunction—present and future. Urol Clin North Am 1995; 1995:879–885.

108. Broderick G. Changing practice patterns in erectile dysfunction: a diagnostic algorithm for the new millennium. Adv Ren Replace Ther 1999; 6:314–326.

109. Ballard S, Gingell C, Tang K, Turner L, Price M, Naylor A. Effects of sildenafil on the relaxation of human corpus cavernosum tissue in vitro and on the activities of cyclic nucleotide phosphodiesterase isozyme. J Urol 1998; 159:2164–2171.

110. Hong E, Lepor H, McCullough A. Time dependent patient satisfaction with sildenafil for erectile dysfunction (ED) after nerve-sparing radical retropubic prostatectomy (RRP). Int J Impot Res 1999; 11:S15–S22.

111. Eardley I. New oral therapies for the treatment of erectile dysfunction. Br J Urol 1998; 81:122–127.

112. Boyce E, Umland E. Sildenafil citrate: a therapeutic update. Clin Ther 2001; 23:2–23.

113. Rendell M, Rajfer J, Wicker P, Smith M. Sildenafil for treatment of erectile dysfunction in men with diabetes: a randomized controlled trial. J Am Med Assoc 1999; 281:421–426.

114. Zippe C, Kedia A, Kedia K, Nelson D, Agarwal A. Treatment of erectile dysfunction after radical prostatectomy with sildenafil citrate (Viagra). Urology 1998; 52:963–966.

115. Derry F, Dinsmore W, Fraser M, Gardner B, Glass C, Maytom M, Smith M. Efficacy and safety of oral sildenafil (Viagra) in men with erectile dysfunction caused by spinal cord injury. Neurology 1998; 51:1629–1633.

116. Stolk E. Cost utility analysis of sildenafil compared to papaverine-phentolamine injection. B Med J 2000; 32:1156–1157.

117. Hatzichristou D, Apostolidis A, Tzortzis V, Ioannides E, Yannakoyorgos K, Kalinderis A. Sildenafil versus intracavernous injection therapy: efficacy and preference in patients on intracavernous injection for more than one year. J Urol 2000; 164:1197–1200.

118. Giuliano F, Montorsi F, Mirone V, Rossi D, Sweeney M. Switching from intracavernous prostaglandin E1 injections to oral sildenafil citrate in patients with erectile dysfunction: results of a multicenter European study. The Sildenafil Multicenter Study Group. J Urol 2000; 164:708–711.

119. McMahon C, Samali R, Johnson H. Treatment of intracorporeal injection nonresponse with sildenafil alone or in combination with triple agent intracorporeal injection therapy. J Urol 1999; 162:1992–1998.

120. Morales A, Gingell C, Collins M, Wicker P, Osterloh I. Clinical safety of oral sildenafil citrate (VIAGRA) in the treatment of erectile dysfunction. Int J Impot Res 1998; 10:69–73.

121. Price D, Gingell J, Gepi-Attee S, Wareham K, Yates P, Boolell M. Sildenafil: study of a novel oral treatment for erectile dysfunction in diabetic men. Diabet Med 1998; 15:821–825.

122. Kloner R. Cardiovascular risk and sildenafil. Am J Cardiol 2000; 86:57f–61f.

123. Cheitlin M, Hutter AJ, Brindis R, Ganz P, Kaul S, Russell RJ, Zusman R. Use of sildenafil (Viagra) in patients with cardiovascular disease. Circulation 1999; 99:168–177.

124. Choi H, Seong D, Rha K. Clinical efficacy of Korean red ginseng for erectile dysfunction. Int J Impot Res 1995; 7:181–186.

125. Costabile R, Spevak M. Oral trazadone is not effective therapy for erectile dysfunction: a double-blind, placebo controlled trial. J Urol 1999; 161:1819–1822.

126. Mulhall J, Goldstein I. Oral agents in the management of erectile dysfunction. In: Carson C, Kirby R, Goldstein I, eds. Textbook of Erectile Dysfunction. Oxford: ISIS Medical Media, 1999;309–315.

127. Meinhardt W, Schmitz P, Kropman R, de la Fuente R, Lycklama a Nijeholt A, Zwartendijk J. Trazadone, a double blind trial for treatment of erectile dysfunction. Int J Impot Res 1997; 9:163–165.

128. Ernst E, Pittler M. Yohimbine for erectile dysfunction: a systematic review and meta-analysis of randomized clinical trials. J Urol 1998; 159:433–436.

129. Kunelius P, Hakkinen J, Lukkarinen O:Is high-dose yohimbine hydrochloride effective in the treatment of mixed-type impotence? A prospective, randomized, controlled double-blind crossover study. Urology 1997; 49:441–444.

130. Teloken C, Rhoden E, Sogari P, Dambros M, Souto C. Therapeutic effects of high dose yohimbine hydroclide on organic erectile dysfunction. J Urol 1998; 159:122–124.

131. Carson C. erectile dysfunction: diagnosis and management with newer oral agents. Baylor Univ Med Cent Proc 2000; 13:356–360.

132. Zorgniotti A. Experience with buccal phentolamine mesylate for impotence. Int J Impot Res 1994; 6:37–41.

133. Becker A, Steif C, Machtens S, Schultheiss D, Hartmann U, Truss M, Jonas U. Oral phentolamine as treatment for erectile dysfunction. J Urol 1998; 159:1214–1216.

134. Goldstein I, Carson C, Rosen R, Islam A. Vasomax for the treatment of male erectile dysfunction. World J Urol 2001; 19:51–56.

135. Gonzales-Cadavid N, Rajfer J. Future therapeutic alternatives in the treatment of erectile dysfunction. In: Carson C, Kirby R, Goldstein I, eds. Textbook of Erectile Dysfunction. Oxford: ISIS Medical Media, 1999; 355–364.
136. Zorgniotti A, Lizza E. Effect of large doses of the nitric oxide precursor, L-arginine, on erectile dysfunction. Int J Impot Res 1994; 6:33–36.
137. Meinhardt W, Kropman R, Vermeij P. Comparative tolerability and efficacy of treatments for impotence. Drug Saf 1999; 20:133–146.
138. Heaton J. Apomorphine: an update of clinical trial results. Int J Impot Res 2000; 12:S67–S73
139. Young J, Auerbauh S, Porst H. Vardenafil, a new selective PDE5 inhibitor, significantly improved all IIEF domains and showed a favorable safety profile in patients with erectile dysfunction over 12 weeks. J Urol 2001; 165:924A.
140. Padma-Nathan H, Rosen R, Shabsigh R, Saikali K, Watkins V, Pullman B. Cialis (IC351) provides prompt response and extended period of responsiveness for the treatment of men with erectile dysfunction (ED). J Urol 2001; 165:923A.

Index